Praise for *When What Gives Way to Why*

Rebecca Claeys lays out a relatable lived experience that hit deeply and connected with my own impractical sense of what work has seemingly evolved into. I've lived it as well.

Doreen Durka, Author of **Lost and Found**

A beautiful book that reignites a fire in your belly to reach for what you really want. It's a step-by-step return journey to your authentic self by way of your own personal hot mess of anxiety and burnout.

Nicole Washburn, Author of **Copywriting Magic** and **Creative Magic**

I value Rebecca's honest and straightforward voice as she shares truths that resonate with me on a deep level. Her encouragement to seek personal value beyond productivity is right on the mark. Leaning into the discomfort of growth and pulling in community around you are themes I am passionate about and I'm thrilled to see Rebecca's bold statements in these areas. This is an insightful book that belongs on your shelf.

CA Jalonen, Author of **Liminal Life**

A fresh take on an OLD problem. It is so much more than a recovery strategy for burnout. It is about living a life that allows for so much more. The perfect accompaniment for anyone looking for a solution to feeling stuck in a hamster wheel life.

Darlene Turriff, Author of Mastering the Protocol and The 4 Soulpreneur Agreements

❧

When What Gives Way to Why opened my eyes to why I've suffered physically from over-achieving throughout my life. Rebecca Claeys helped me to see that the drive to always be productive actually takes away from our purpose (and joy). This book will help you make a mindset shift that will quickly move you from burnout to putting focus on the actions that will truly bring you joy in life.

Maria Brophy, Author of Art Money Success and Empowered Women's Circle

❧

Detaching from the expected hustle of society and finding ourselves is at the core of ***When What Gives Way to Why***. This book is empowering, helps reframe much of how we see life and work, and gives us the tools and exercises to start creating inner change.

Lara Wellman, Author of You're Not Lazy

When What Gives Way to Why

when
WHAT
gives
way
to
WHY

Rebecca Claeys

Author: Claeys, Rebecca
Title: When What Gives Way to Why
ISBN: 979-8-9890352-3-6

Editors: Nicole Washburn, Darlene Turiff
Cover Art: Sanna Nilsson
Photography Credit: Maeve Turner-Johnson

Reddig Relationship Circles Model © 2022 Jennifer Reddig, MSW, LICSW, CCTP
Used with permission

Published by Cleopatra's Seeds, LLC
Spring Green, WI
www.cleopatrasseeds.com

*Dedicated with utmost love to
Mary Margaret Cathers,
the first person to see - and
celebrate - my core self.*

Author's Note

Writing this book has been a labor of love, borne from a workshop series and a challenging journey through burnout to my own healing. It's not a light book because healing doesn't come from bypassing the heavy stuff in our lives. We find it by addressing it head on through solid, steady work.

I've never been a fan of bypassing or 'good enough' solutions. I want things that I invest my energy into fixing to stay fixed. After all, if I can't take the time to do it right the first time, when will I be able to find the time to fix it again?

If you're looking for that same kind of healing, the kind that doesn't crumble at the slightest sign of stress, this is the book for you. It *will* take work. Only you can do that work. That's where the payoff is, though - the more earnest your intention is as you complete the exercises throughout the book, the stronger your foundation of healing will be. Nobody will be able to take that away from you.

I also want to recognize the significant privilege I have in writing this book and in addressing my burnout.

As a white, middle class, female-presenting person, there are opportunities and considerations afforded to me that I have not earned. There are also struggles I am unaware of simply because I have not had to face them, nor have I learned about them from others.

I am working to decolonize my mind and heart, expose myself to the daily challenges of my fellow humans, and use the privilege I have been afforded to minimize the impacts of systemic injustice wherever I can. I am still learning. I will make mistakes; I likely have made a few in this book. I will continue to adjust my language and approach as I learn more, and am grateful for grace given as I work to correct my errors.

Thank you for coming on this journey with me. It won't be a simple one, and you'll never be alone on it.

With endless gratitude,

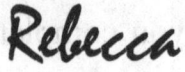

TABLE OF CONTENTS

Introduction 1

1 Crashing and Learning 11

2 Your Personal Key 27

3 Gardens and Villages 35

    Exercise 1: Creature Comforts 42

    Exercise 2: Find Your Village 46

4 The B Word 55

    Exercise 3: Releasing the Burden 64

    Exercise 4: Letting Go 70

5 Grammar's Cool 83

6 What vs. Why 93

    Exercise 5: Spring Cleaning 98

7 Finding Yourself 107

    Exercise 6: Field Notes 117

8 Threads Make the Tapestry 121

    Exercise 7: Investigation 125

    Exercise 8: Analysis 128

    Exercise 9: Distillation 130

    Exercise 10: Naming Your Why 132

9 Here Be Dragons 139

    Exercise 11: Haven Sweet Haven 142

    Exercise 12: Your Personal Treasure Map 148

    Exercise 13: Rituals Are Not Luxuries 159

10 Into Your Unknown 163

Acknowledgements 173

INTRODUCTION

When was the last time you weren't tired? I'm talking about that bone-deep tired that you can't describe, sleep won't fix, and you're pretty sure nobody else has ever felt. Close your eyes and think back. Was it before a relationship? Was it before you became a parent? Was it before you entered the workforce? Was it when you were still a child?

We use the words 'burned out' as either a misplaced badge of honor or a chronic personal descriptor in our culture. Especially coming out of the COVID-19 pandemic, it seems like everyone is burned out, and nobody has a good answer on how to stop. Can you remember a time before you were burned out? Or have you always been? What would your life look like if burnout wasn't mandatory?

1

The burnout/purpose industry that has been built up to capitalize on our overwhelm uses a lot of words to define burnout, describing one basic effect: you've become disconnected from your work and your productivity. You no longer feel capable of achieving what you think you should. This disconnection, the experts in this industry hypothesize, bleeds into other areas of your life and causes increasing amounts of stress. Stress is the target for this industry: get rid of stress, and you'll be right back to your old self in no time.

Industry-standard treatment revolves around reducing your stressors, relaxing, and getting you to a place where you can once again connect to your work and become productive. Take a vacation to an airy villa just off a tropical beach or a cozy cabin in the woods. Get yourself some retail therapy - treat yourself to some new candles or that gorgeous pair of beaded sandals staring at you through a storefront window. Do some self-care at home for a quick hit of dopamine (a long, luxurious bath sounds nice, maybe with those candles you just bought and the bougie bath bomb at the register that you couldn't resist).

From a societal standpoint, these tactics make complete sense. The goal of treatment is returning to productivity because in this society, your personal worth is tied to how much you can produce. You feel good in the moment of indulging in rest like you've been able to struggle to the surface of the ocean and take a mighty gulp of new, clean air. After suffocating for so long, that singular breath may make you feel like you can take on the world.

These strategies to address burnout are a temporary respite from the stressors though; they're waiting for you when you get back. The bills don't disappear because you went on vacation. Work emails with demands that apparently only you can fulfill don't stop piling up in your absence. The doctor appointments and the music lessons, and sports practices all still exist and need to be managed.

Even the bougiest bath bomb can't wash away the multitude of equally important tasks vying for your attention and energy. That gulp of air is enough to keep you alive when you get pulled back under the surface, but it is not enough to sustain you. You soon begin suffocating again.

Frankly, a lot of your stressors may follow you on your vacations or self-care rituals, like waves slapping you in the face while you're trying to pull in that full breath of life-sustaining air. Despite your best intentions, they invade your mind as guilt and shame for stepping away or an irresistible draw to just 'check in with the office' to make sure everything isn't imploding. Is there anything less relaxing than planning out your schedule for your return to the office in the middle of a massage or a bit of family time on the beach?

The tie of productivity to your worth in the world is so strong that it has become the subconscious equivalent of a weight around your ankles, pulling you back into the deep. If you aren't productive as much as you can be whenever you can be, you become unworthy, or at least less worthy.

We offer our health and personal happiness as a sacrifice at the altar of productivity in the hopes of being affirmed in our worth.

You become less deserving of the nice things in life. Status, with the accompanying social benefits, lies out of reach. Leisure is wasteful because that is time you could be spending being productive. Side hustles, anyone? What hobby have you monetized because you could, at the very least, enjoy the productivity while you tried to bring in a bit more money? Did you end up hating that hobby? Did you actually make any money from it?

Everyone is burned out because nobody has a good answer on how to stop. The answers that are front-and-center are ones necessarily rooted in the problem: the myth of productivity. This idea of producing all of the time everywhere is a foundation of our society. By tying personal worth to productivity, we willingly accept the need to continually produce to prove our worthiness, no matter the cost to ourselves or those around us. We offer our health and personal happiness as a sacrifice at the altar of productivity in the hopes of being affirmed in our worth.

Society encourages us to keep pushing, keep producing by handing out accolades for productivity, whether that's an award for completing a project, a promotion, or the quintessential watch or coffee mug for longevity with an organization. Seeing your colleagues receive these tokens is supposed to incentivize you to work harder, do more, better, faster. Surely, you'll be recognized for your hard work and will be rewarded too! If you're not recognized, you're simply not working hard enough.

This, of course, is by design. These gold-plated handcuffs promise you that more is just around the corner if you only keep going. But of course, the corner never ends because it's a circle. This culture, this behavior, is normalized. We accept it because there is nothing else we've ever known. It's just how life is.

What if life didn't have to be that way? What if you had the opportunity to just *be* with no expectations, no guilt, no pressure, and no goals? What if your success wasn't measured by how much you produce but by how much your actions align with your values? What if you owned the key to unlock your own gold-plated handcuffs, and you've just been taught not to look for it where it actually lives?

What if that key not only unlocks your handcuffs but opens the door to a more fulfilled, complete life that you and you alone get to design? A life where, instead of struggling for gulps of air above the ocean surface, you've walked out of the ocean and can breathe freely, choosing when and where to dip back into the water. In this life, you're not waiting for someone to hand you an award. You've already decided what success looks like, and you are the one who decides when you're there.

There's no more circle to push around. You can go in any direction you'd like because your goal is not producing more; it's ensuring your life is in alignment with your core values. You have drawn the map of your journey based on what matters to you, yourself, without outside interference. You can make changes to your map through decisions about challenges and opportunities with certainty because you have a framework that you have built to guide you. You are in control, and the grace and ease with which you move through life radiates off of you like a thousand shooting stars.

What if I told you this life is possible, and I can show you where that key lives?

nigredo

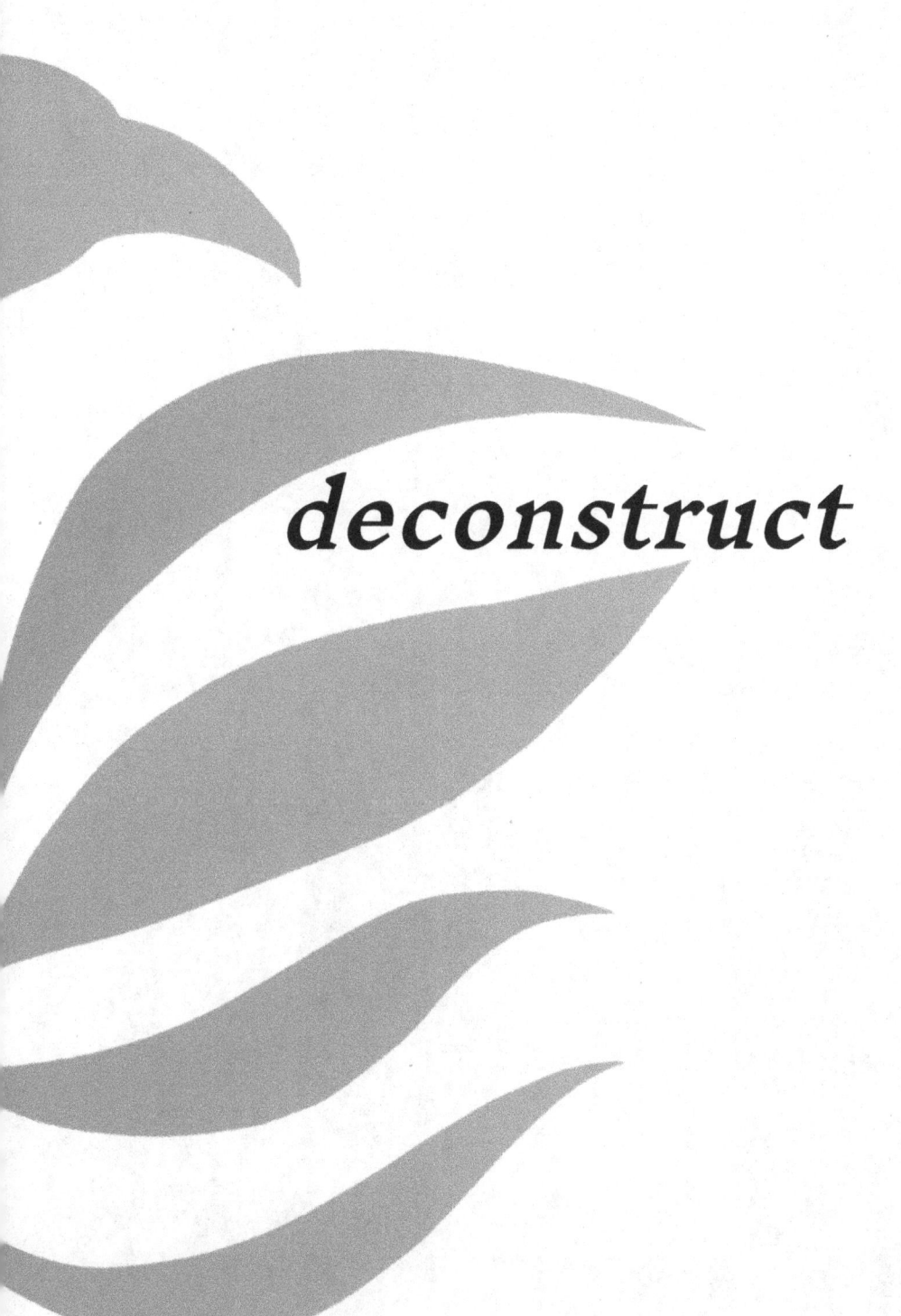

deconstruct

1

CRASHING AND LEARNING

When I woke up and logged in to my work computer on the morning of May 19, 2020, I had no idea that my life was about to completely change.

I was thoroughly content with my 5-foot commute from my bed to my desk and was really settling into this new mode of working. No more getting up at 5 a.m. to get myself ready and out the door by 5:45 so I could commute an hour or more through heavy traffic into a government office building, only to finish a long day and commute another hour or more through heavier traffic home. Five years of tailored trousers, eye-catching blouses, and structured blazers had been traded in for "soft pants" and long sleeved t-shirts that were smooth and soft as butter, and I was reveling in the newfound comfort of my work-from-home setup.

Nestled into my brand new ergonomic chair, I had my daily cup of coffee in hand and was running my standard morning reports to assess the new federal policy changes inspired by the COVID-19 pandemic that impacted Medicaid. My work unit would use this information to understand how to oversee Medicaid providers across our state, ensuring that vulnerable people would have access to high-quality medical care at a time they needed it the most. Even though I wasn't using my RN license to work on the front lines of the pandemic, I was still making a difference in the lives of people around me. My work had meaning.

About two hours into my day, I received an email from the Inspector General, four layers of management above me. The Secretary's Office needed volunteers to work at the State Emergency Operations Center on the statewide pandemic response. They were looking for a four to six week commitment, and I had to decide by the end of the work day because I would have to report to the SEOC the next morning. I was given no other information about what I would be doing, equipment I should bring with me, or who I would connect with when I arrived there. I was simply asked to show up, and it didn't feel much like not volunteering was an option.

My family had been cloistered in our home for two months at this point, very careful to avoid all but the most necessary in-person interaction. I was absolutely terrified at the thought of being amongst a hundred strangers for a month or more. We still didn't understand enough about how COVID-19 spread, how to accurately screen for it, or what precautions were necessary to prevent its spread. It felt like I was being volunteered to go into a well-lit plague house dressed with silks and lace. I could potentially bring home a disease that could severely impact my family, and I would have no idea I'd done it.

At the same time, this was a huge opportunity for me professionally. I had been stuck in a rut in my role within the Office of the Inspector General and was chafing at the limits I worked under. In this assignment, I would be working shoulder-to-shoulder with the top echelon of staff and management within the Department of Health Services. I'd have the opportunity to build relationships and show other people what kind of work I was capable of. I felt honored to be included in that group, and the thought of being included in such an adept and accomplished group also awakened that monster so many of us are familiar with: imposter syndrome.

Was I actually good enough to be a peer of these people? Could I hack it, especially in such a high-pressure environment? There had to be a reason I'd been chosen for this; someone thought my work - my ability - measured up to this group. It was hard for me to see and harder for me to accept.

I sipped my coffee (that some might mistake for iced, but I knew from daily practice that it was chilled through distraction and neglect) and discussed the situation with my ever-patient husband. He encouraged me to take the leap and try it out despite the potential exposure to our family. He knew the limits in my work environment agitated me. He wanted to see me recognized for my skills and efforts.

With his prodding, I took a deep breath and sent my acceptance. I then promptly freaked out about whether my tailored trousers would still fit, because I was pretty sure frayed and stained yoga pants did not meet the dress code.

The next morning, I was up at 5. The old routine came back with a bit of a struggle. I left the house only a little bit late and made my way to a red brick building that, were it not for the military guard at the entrance, might be mistaken for a tech startup office. I swallowed the lump in my throat and produced my employee ID, only to be anticlimactically waved through into the parking lot.

I walked inside and followed some hastily created signs on printer paper to a room where I would have a temporal thermometer waived at me by a uniformed National Guard member. When I registered as normal, I received a small colored card stamped with the date to display on the back side of my ID. I'd soon build a small collection of these colored cards as a new one in a different color was needed each day to prove that I'd been cleared by not having a fever.

After wandering around the maze of the building for about twenty minutes (I must have looked purposeful because nobody questioned me), I found myself in a large 'situation room' like you would see on TV shows. The giant screen on the back wall and floor filled with rows of desks was intimidating and surreal. How had I ended up in this place? People like me didn't operate in places like this one. Surely there was a mistake. Doubt filled me and sat like a pit in my stomach for the entire day, despite the warm welcome I received from the team lead I'd be working under. I resolved to dig in and use what skills I had, however I could.

Of course, the four to six weeks I'd agreed to was extremely optimistic in hindsight. As we approached that first marker, I had been pulled fully into the work and was juggling multiple roles within the team. When asked if I wanted to continue the work, I enthusiastically said yes! My work with Medicaid had meaning. This work had *purpose*. I was directly impacting the pandemic and people's lives. We could measure it. It was incredibly rewarding to be a part of this amazing team and to see the fruits of my labor play out on a daily basis.

After six months, I was extended again. By this point, I'd taken over the new electronic test registration and results delivery software and was working on getting it established at testing sites across the state. I was deemed too instrumental to the work to let go - not that I really wanted to go back. I felt a freedom and autonomy here I'd rarely experienced in my professional life, and I didn't want to let it go. Six months stretched into a year. And then fifteen months. And then eighteen. Every challenge that came to me, I conquered with my team.

I was now leading a team of 24 and actively involved in the development of a more permanent piece of software to facilitate testing. The work we were doing was being moved into the permanent structure of the department, and I was hired into the supervisor role over the unit responsible for the new software's management. By all accounts, I had made it. I was successful. I was productive and had accomplishments and awards and honors to show for everything I'd poured into this response.

And I was broken.

I had been working 60-70 hour weeks for eighteen months straight because it was necessary. I did not have days off. I was always on call. Before I started building my team, I was technical support, operational support, data support, communications, and administration for my software. The work never had a break because viruses don't take weekends or holidays off. I was exhausted and unfulfilled. It didn't matter that I had all of the accolades I'd garnered throughout the response or statistics to support my success. I was burned out beyond burned out.

17

Now that I was in a more permanent role and had a team to take some of the work off of me, I tried to address my burnout. I knew I couldn't keep on in the state I was in, so I tapped into that burnout-purpose industry that is so ubiquitous and tried all of the usual solutions.

I talked about it with my therapist. I read so, so many books. I listened to more podcasts on burnout than I can remember. I watched videos of experts on the subject talking in 15-20 minute increments on how to beat burnout. Every single one came down to "take a vacation and don't stress so much." As if it's that easy.

I'd always found a way to beat any challenge life had thrown my way before - why couldn't I cut it this time?

I tried all of the methods I could get my hands on, and some of them actually helped – for three days. And then I was right back to the misery and hopelessness that exemplified my burnout. Nothing was working. I felt like a failure because I couldn't beat this. I'd always found a way to beat any challenge life had thrown my way before - why couldn't I cut it this time? I was convinced that I was permanently damaged by this work that I had sacrificed so much of myself already for. The virus hadn't gotten me, but the response absolutely had.

When I started working with my therapist, I viewed the entire pandemic response experience as if it was a half-blended fruit smoothie: occasional chunks of frozen strawberry or banana popped out when you weren't expecting them, but it was mostly a uniform experience. The more we talked, though, the easier it was for me to realize that there were clear segments with very different mindsets, emotional environments, and limitations.

Exploring those segments and how they impacted my physical and mental health was critical to my understanding of burnout and my eventual climb out of it. It wasn't an overnight journey by any means. Now, though, I've gathered that journey and all of the labor that went into it, so you can also benefit from what I've learned.

The single most impactful point of clarity that came to me was that the cause of burnout wasn't adequately defined by those books, podcasts, or experts with internet videos. My nursing education kicked in here: if

19

you don't understand the underlying cause, you'll only be treating symptoms. If your assessment isn't thorough enough, you will miss essential context clues that allow you to develop a plan to treat the condition. This is why those methods only lasted three days at most; they were treating symptoms rather than addressing the systemic issues that create those symptoms.

If you look around and talk to more than a handful of people, you will notice that just about everyone around you is stressed. They are tired. They work too hard, too much, and get too little in return. This is certainly concentrated at the lower end of the socioeconomic spectrum and heavily weighted by race and gender, and those who seem to have all of the outward signs of success in the world are not immune. Our societal systems are set up in such a way that we all experience excessive fatigue, overwork, and plateaus of not-enoughness. These are symptoms. There are thousands more.

How much any one person is weighed down by these barriers - barriers that are imposed on each of us by societal structures - is heavily dependent on the privileges they carry. Privileges are simply characteristics you have, by birth or circumstance, that give you an advantage in societal interactions. The fewer you have, the more likely you are to be impacted by structural inequity, and with greater force. When the lack of privileges piles up, the effect is exponential.

Are you white? If so, you are less likely to be impacted than your black and brown neighbors, all other things being equal. Are you a woman or female-presenting? Society has dictated that women, or those it perceives as women, should bear the mental and emotional labor in a household in addition to any professional labor they perform. When, for example, race and gender overlap, they meld together to bring about an entirely new set of expectations, pressures, and privilege differentials to navigate.

Your worth lies in being you, as fully and wholly as you possibly can be, even and especially when you produce absolutely nothing.

These are a glimpse of the tip of the iceberg into privilege and intersectionality, and there are many wonderful books written by people much more informed than I on the subject that are very worthwhile to fold into your knowledge. I share it here because privileges and how they intersect play an important role in understanding where I believe, based on my journey, burnout actually originates from.

We'll dig into that more deeply in a little while. Right now, the important part for you to remember is that you are a human being, not a human doing. These societal structures I've mentioned stress the need to be productive so much that we have learned from a young age to tie our personal worth to how much we produce. I promise you, this is not where your worth lies. Your worth lies in being you, as fully and wholly as you possibly can be, even and especially when you produce absolutely nothing.

It's easy for me to say that, right? I'm not paying your bills. I'm not feeding your family, worrying about cupcakes that need to be baked for school last minute, getting the dog to the vet for that weird limp that showed up out of nowhere, mowing your lawn (or plowing your driveway, depending on where you live and what time of year it is). I'm not doing your job and dealing with your boss and coworkers day in and day out. I'm not under your deadlines, myriad as they are. I don't carry your daily load of all of the tasks that nobody seems to notice.

You're here because you're tired. You've tried the books, the podcasts, the internet videos, the supplements, and the exercise programs. Nothing has helped for more than a couple of days or a couple of weeks at most.

Take a moment and think about how you would spend your time if you had no obligations and money was no object. How would your day flow? Is your instinct to think about all of the things you could accomplish, or are you more focused on how you would exist in your environment? Is it a mix of both? Which is weighted more heavily? Most importantly, would your answer actually bring you to a place of peace and contentment?

I won't promise you a miracle cure with this book, because if there was a miracle cure, everyone would take it. What I will promise is that by the end of this book, if you follow through all of the exercises and walk this journey with me, you will have a radically different view of yourself and your life. This book will walk you through developing a new mindset for viewing your world, one based on your values rather than on the priorities others put on you. It will help you build a framework for making decisions as you move through life that will leave you more satisfied with your choices.

By the time you turn the last page, you will understand not only how to deal with the symptoms coming at you every day, but how to finally, finally treat that underlying cause. You will be able to see a path forward toward joy – a path that is lined with peace and contentment, ready for you to embrace.

2

Your Personal Key

If you do an internet search for the phrase "personal purpose," you'll retrieve upwards of 3.7 billion results. That's a lot of results. This displays very clearly and simply the fascination humanity has with bringing meaning to our individual lives. We want to know that there is a reason for our existence, that we as individuals have an impact on the world around us. Existential crises are nothing new, and industries have been built around helping people find the meaning of their singular life.

A brief perusal of the top returns in these 3.7 billion results reads like a how-to on mirroring your life to a company's structure. Your personal purpose statement should define your goals, they claim. It should explain what you want to accomplish in life. It should elaborate on why you get out of bed in the morning, inspire positive change, and keep you focused on the future. While you're at it, you should write a mission and vision statement to go along with them! Sounds pretty good, doesn't it? It works well for companies, so it should work well for you. This handful of statements should give you everything you need to understand why you exist and keep you moving into the future!

Of course, you and I both know that this is nonsense. You're not a company; you're a human being. You can't run yourself like a company because a company is not a sentient individual. It doesn't have the depth and complexity that you have. It is one thing, while you are many things to many people.

Because you are a human being, you have purpose. Not a purpose, but purpose. It is granted to you simply by existing.

The relationships you develop are so much more nuanced than a company's could ever be. The reason you exist is orders of magnitude more intricate than a company's reason for existence. You are *not* a company, and you should never try to pretend you are. You are a human being.

Because you are a human being, you have purpose. Not a purpose, but purpose. It is granted to you simply by existing. You don't have to earn it. You don't have to craft it. You simply have it. You receive it the moment you take your first breath in the world, and you carry it with you until you take your last.

Uncovering that purpose, understanding it, and living it is a different story. As with anything valuable in our lives, understanding your purpose will take some work. This work takes more effort when you've been taught that your purpose is not an integral part of who you are, but what you produce.

Western culture emphatically ingrains in our minds that we must produce. If you don't produce something that contributes to society, you are less valuable to those around you. You are less worthy of having resources. You are less worthy of attention and investment of skill and energy.

Conversely, the more you produce, the more worthy you become. You receive praise, awards, promotions, and raises. Your public profile becomes higher. You become someone who people want to be around and be like. The investment of time, skill, and energy that people willingly give you becomes almost limitless. Even low levels of fame become attractive and desirable because that's when your acknowledgment of your own personal worth is socially appropriate.

This mindset insists that you operate as a machine if you are to be honored. Human-driven manufacturing has shifted from factories to skyscrapers, from assembly lines to cube farms. People are measured like machines, compared to fabricated metrics nominally based on how much output they create. Comparing yourself to a machine has become a flex.

Even in a post-pandemic world where work from home has become more normalized, there is a drive to increase production. If you're not productive enough at home, you're threatened with going back to the cube farm. Alternatively, the learned compulsion to act as a machine kicks in: you don't have to commute or spend as much time getting ready in the morning, so you may as well spend that extra time getting a bit more cranked out, right?

This reads like an incredibly bleak, dystopian existence. And yet, it is what we have all agreed to as a culture. You and I, as individuals, have collectively, subconsciously, and by tradition, chosen to buy into this broad social agreement because of the mirage of success that comes along with it. The mirage brings an outward level of comfort and regard, but it can never bring inward peace or contentment. The only thing that will ever meet that base human need is alignment with your purpose.

Your purpose, that intangible key that unlocks the door to true freedom, is in your possession. It's been tucked away on a hidden shelf because you have been taught that it has no place in 'adult' life. It's one of those childish things that you were told you needed to mature past so you could make it in the world. Ultimately, embracing your purpose is the most 'adult' thing you can do because it forces you to question everything you've been told and everything you see around you. It demands you acknowledge that you are a human being, not a human doing.

Your purpose is a beacon, powered by those things you hold most dear, that illuminates what is truly important in your life. Its light is so intense that the mirages in your life will burn into oblivion, leaving only a small pile of ash as if a phoenix had been reborn. Your values drive it. Your existence fulfills it. Your joy affirms it. It is no wonder you were taught to keep it hidden away; can you imagine the power you would wield if you fully embraced it?

To get there, you will have to rebuild yourself to a degree, like a phoenix about to regenerate. You will need to deconstruct what you think you know, purify your language around it, transmute your beliefs, and rebuild your reality. I named this process the Soul Alchemy Cycle. As you work through this book, you will find yourself walking through each phase of the cycle, even though you may not immediately recognize it as such. I'll be there, walking alongside you, matching you step for step.

This process won't be an easy or a comfortable one. In fact, a big part of it is getting uncomfortable intentionally. You can't rebuild yourself if you're not willing to go through some changes. Change is not comfortable; just ask the phoenix.

Remember, though, that this change is about you. You aren't changing the world around you; you are changing how you move through it. This book is not about how to quit your job, make your spouse a better person, or make people appreciate the amazing being you are. It's not about saving the world.

I'm not saying those things can't happen or won't be an end result after you've worked through the Cycle. I'm simply saying that this book is not about those 'what' things. It's about *why* you choose *what* you choose. Understand the why – understand *your* why – and claim what has always been yours.

3

GARDENS AND VILLAGES

Before we can dive into the really hard work, you need to spend some time shifting your mindset. Approaching this method without getting in the right headspace will provide limited benefit because the method is all about shifting perspective and operating from a new way of thinking. Right now is the perfect time to practice this skill – letting go of what *should* be and leaning into what *is*, seeing your world and your life through a different window frame, even if it's only five feet to the right or left.

This is not a natural skill for most humans. We all develop neural connections as shortcuts to make our brains do less work. These shortcuts are like the expressway: straightforward and easy to find. It takes a lot of conscious effort to refuse to get on the expressway and take the scenic route.

Navigating winding roads using a paper map, minimal road signs, and our own sense of direction is challenging and so very much more rewarding than simply using the same fast route that we've always used. So come on this winding journey with me, even if it doesn't always make sense, and let's enjoy the beauty around us.

Unpot Yourself

I'm an amateur gardener. I'll admit my thumbs aren't the greenest, and I've picked up a few things over the years through trial and error (mostly error). Living in the great frozen north, we have a much shorter growing season than much of humanity. This means we need to give plants a boost by starting seeds indoors, in a climate-controlled environment that mimics the warmth and moisture of spring and encourages growth.

When starting a plant indoors, it's typically in a small container only slightly larger than a grown man's thumb. This is because we start a lot of seeds at once to ensure that we have enough adequately strong plants to survive and produce food into the summer and autumn. We start off knowing that not every seed we plant will survive or thrive, and we accept that. Regardless, we're going to give each plant every opportunity possible to become strong and thriving.

Imagine with me that we've planted a tomato seed in a starter container. There are probably two tablespoons of soil in that container for one seed to grow into, plenty for a good start. Our seed sprouts and starts growing a nice, sturdy stem and big, beautiful leaves. First, the primary leaves, and then the secondary and tertiary sets emerge. The unmistakable scent of a tomato plant starts to fill the air around it, bright and slightly spicy.

The stem grows taller to give these leaves room to expand and create more food for our baby plant. As the stem grows, so too do the roots, deep into our two tablespoons of soil. Soon, those branching roots reach the bottom of the starter container and start to wrap themselves around what soil there is. Our plant is becoming root-bound.

If we leave our tomato plant in the starter container, it will quickly use up the nutrients in that small amount of soil and begin to digest itself in an attempt to stay alive. Our only alternative to keep it thriving is to transplant it. If it's still too early to plant outside, we can move it to a larger container and give it more room to grow while keeping it protected. If the weather outside has warmed enough to not endanger this tender plant even at night, we can move it directly into the dirt outside. Either way, it needs to be disturbed and moved.

Now, our plant likes its starter container. It knows where the boundaries are. It knows how to gather the nutrients it needs. It is comfortable in this place, even though it cannot survive here long term. It would rather not be moved because this is the only home it has ever known. We know, however, that it must be moved if it is to have a chance of surviving and thriving.

That means we have to pull it out of the starter container. We need to loosen the roots so they have the ability to expand and grow in new ways in its new home. This is very, very uncomfortable for the plant. Familiarity is gone. Boundaries are gone. It can't follow the old way of doing things because it doesn't have the same infrastructure it had before. But once we tenderly bury its roots in its new home and gently blanket them with fresh soil, maybe even with some compost mixed in for an extra boost of goodies, it has a chance.

Our now preteen plant is going to be grumpy (I know I would be - you might be too, and that's ok! Change is a hard thing, and you can do hard things.) It is going to act out a bit for the first couple days. It needs extra nurturing, nourishing, and encouragement to establish itself in its new home so it can figure out how to start stretching its roots back out and building a new infrastructure on which it can thrive.

Be willing, throughout this process and throughout your life, to unpot yourself.

We, as caring gardeners, give it a bit of extra water. We may talk to it about how well it's doing, praise it for its growth and adjustment. We pay close attention to its needs and listen to what it tells us it's missing so we can support it and provide resources through this adjustment period. Sometimes, we make mistakes in our understanding of what it needs; we give ourselves grace as caretakers and shift strategies.

And eventually, it takes off. Our plant now digs deep with its roots and drinks up all of the good stuff we provide it. We may have to go through this unpotting process several times to make sure our plant is growing in the best possible environment before it lands in its final home. We do this with each plant as an individual, knowing that these are living entities and they grow at their own paces, with different needs on different timelines.

Gardening is a lot like tending ourselves. We, too, are living entities that grow at our own pace, with needs and timelines that differ from others around us. We start in a stable place that allows us to develop our root structure, but we may quickly outgrow that place and become root-bound. Be willing, throughout this process and throughout your life, to unpot yourself. Get uncomfortable, because discomfort is the path to growth.

Remember to nourish yourself, listen to what your body and mind are asking for, and give yourself grace if you don't get it right the first time. You are both the plant and the gardener, which is a lot of responsibility to shoulder. You *are* strong enough to handle both roles.

Collect Your Gardening Tools

It's easy for me to tell you to nourish yourself. It's a lot harder to discern what you actually need to do to accomplish that goal. Before you dive into the journey ahead, take the opportunity to fill your gardening bag with tools that will help you tend to yourself.

As you progress through this exercise, as well as all other exercises in this book, log your answers however makes sense for you. I'm a write-in-the-book person, but if you prefer a piece of paper, you can hang on the fridge or a journal, those are wonderful too. If you are a spreadsheet jockey or enjoy using another electronic means of recording, by all means, have at it. This method centers you, and that includes tapping into how you best store and receive information. You can also find quick, easy worksheets for this exercise and many others on my website.

Exercise 1: Creature Comforts

Find a quiet spot where you won't be interrupted for 20-30 minutes. Grab your preferred logging method and go through each of the following prompts.

❦ What makes you feel alive?

❦ When you are hurting, do you need social connection to heal, or do you prefer to keep to yourself?

    ❦ Are you somewhere in between?

    ❦ Are there certain people that recharge you and others who drain you?

❦ What is your favorite scent?

❦ What scent(s) do you need to avoid?

❦ What food makes you feel energized and ready to conquer the world?

❧ Do you need movement to feel like yourself?

   ❧ What kind?

   ❧ What intensity?

❧ If you had a week with no responsibilities and no budget limits, what would you do?

   ❧ Where would you go, and who would you visit or take with you?

❧ Does music soothe your mind, energize you, or irritate you?

   ❧ How do different types of music impact your mood and how your body feels?

❧ What textures feel good on your skin?

❧ What textures do you need to avoid at all costs?

Did you notice that many of these prompts are directly related to sensory input? Others are related to stress management, and others to fostering joy. How did it feel to work through this exercise? What did you notice in your body as you were answering the questions? Did you skip it because it felt like too much?

Don't feel ashamed if your answer to that last question is yes. These exercises can be heavy and aren't always the kind of thing you can complete in one sitting. Give yourself some grace and come back to it when you're in a better place to do so. The words on the paper, screen, or audio file aren't going anywhere, nor is the support I'm offering you here. Be gentle with your plant.

All of the concepts embedded in these questions are important when you're identifying how your inner plant needs tending to. Some may be more helpful in a given situation than others, which is why identifying the answers before you undergo discomfort is necessary. You are filling your bag with gardening tools right now so you can tap into it when you are feeling the stress of change and don't have the brain power to decide on something that can help.

When your inner tomato plant is feeling stressed, dig through your gardening bag. Move on instinct, because your instincts are powerful and excellent leaders when assessing your personal needs. What tool sounds like it will be helpful? Is there one that stands out amongst the others? Are there a couple that you can try? Work through these options, starting with the one that jumps out most. If you're not sure which one does, choose one at random and try it. You may need more than one, or you may get an idea of what would *really* help when you are in the process of trying one or more. Follow that instinct. You know you better than anyone in the world. Trust what you know.

Mistakes are how we learn.

You are not going to get this right every time. Trial and error, making mistakes and recovering, are core features of being human. Mistakes are how we learn. Give yourself grace when those mistakes happen. Our learned response in this culture is that mistakes are failures. Setbacks. Proof we aren't good enough. They are marks against our ability to produce reliably.

In reality, they are valuable experiences of what not to do. As long as we take a lesson from our mistakes and choose differently in the future, given the same set of circumstances, we are successful. We are learning. We are human.

We can't always navigate this alone. Unlearning responses is hard. Really, really hard. It takes a lot of time and energy, and it doesn't always leave us with enough to navigate the original issue. This is where your village comes in. Your village consists of the people you trust with the most intimate, vulnerable pieces of you. These may not be the people who immediately come to mind for you. Let's take a moment to assess who lies in your village and who might be in the next village over.

I recently spent some time with Jennifer Reddig, MSW, LICSW, CCTP, to discuss a model she has developed and uses routinely in her practice. The model is all about identifying how people relate to you in your life. It's very helpful for visualizing relationships and the magnitude of their influence on how you live.

Exercise 2: Find Your Village

Keep in mind as you work through this exercise that where someone lands on the model is controlled by their behavior toward you, positive or negative. Nobody inherently gets a specific place on the map because of a role they hold. This map is for you and you alone; be honest in your assessment of these relationships.

One last consideration: children do not belong on this model. We cannot expect them to hold space for us as we would an adult. You can love them very much, with your whole being, and it is kindest for both you and them to leave them off your map.

Step 1:

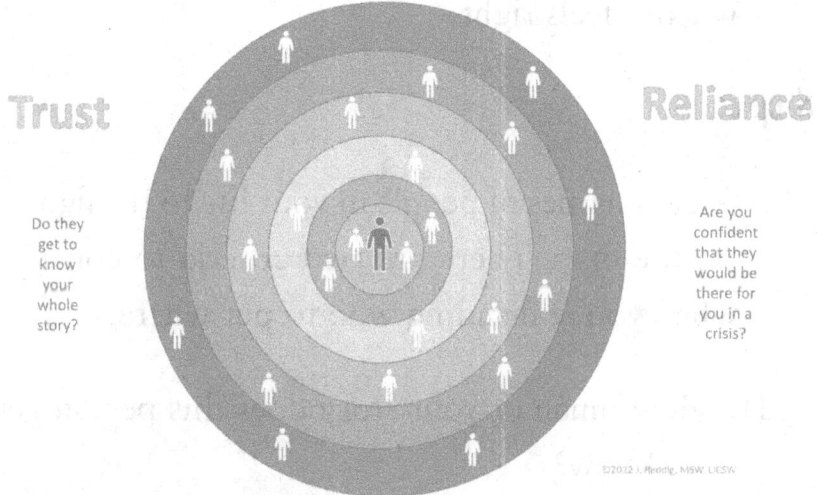

Trust

Do they get to know your whole story?

Reliance

Are you confident that they would be there for you in a crisis?

©2012 J. Meeting, MSW, LICSW

🌿 Draw a set of concentric circles, like a target. Make sure it's big with plenty of room to draw and write on.

🌿 Draw a stick figure that represents you in the bullseye.

47

❦ Draw more stick figures around your target. There may be one or possibly two other figures in the bullseye with you. Other figures are in other circles going out from that center point and may be closer or further from the inner edge of their ring based on how they meet the criteria.

❦ You can have as many or as few circles on your map as feels right to you, and your answer will likely be different from the next person. Stop when it feels right.

Step 2:

❦ Assign names of people in your life to the figures on the map. There are two criteria to consider when you're deciding who to put where.

1) How much of your story does this person get to know?

   ❦ How much of yourself do you trust them with?

   ❦ Are there any aspects of yourself you feel the need to hide around them because they hold power over you?

❧ Do you feel safe sharing the most intimate parts of your identity with them?

2) How much can you depend on this person?

❧ If you were to call this person at 2 a.m. with a flat tire in the middle of nowhere (or you had a different personal crisis), how confident are you that they would drop everything to come help you?

❧ Do you know for certain that you will get help if you ask for it? Don't assume that they would help you because you've helped them. Focus on their historic actions, not your current assumptions.

❧ The people in the bullseye know the most about you, and you are comfortable with sharing anything about yourself freely without fear of judgment. You know without a doubt that they would be there as fast as humanly possible (with or without breaking speed limit laws) to get to you. They are your ride-or-die. Start with those names and work outward.

🌀 Hold each person up to the two criteria and make a decision on which ring, and where in the ring, they belong. There are no right or wrong answers.

How do you know when to stop? Does the guy who drops off your online purchases deserve to live on your map? That's entirely up to you. When you get to a point where you are questioning whether someone belongs on the map or not, sit with their name and pay attention to how you feel in your body. Is there resistance? Listen to it.

You decide how far out your map goes, and you decide who belongs on it. Remember, *nobody*, not even your parent or spouse, has a right to a place on this map because of who they are. They earn it by how they interact with you.

Step 3:

🌀 Once you are content with your map, sit with it. Examine it.

🌀 At which point is there a significant drop-off in either measure?

🍂 If there's not a cliff for either one, at what point does there feel like there is a distance that you wouldn't reach out to for help with a moderate issue (rather than a crisis)?

🍂 Where do you feel like someone knows you, but not well enough to reflect back to you things you can't always see about yourself?

🍂 That point is the boundary of your village. Draw a thick line around it on your map.

Everyone inside that boundary line is in your village. Those who lie outside the line are in neighboring villages. They're very much a part of your life and you may love them deeply. They're not who you are going to depend on when you need help as you work through this process, though. You are going to turn to the people inside your village for that assistance.

Now that you've identified who the members of your village are, you know who to actively foster deeper relationships with. These are the people to ask for help when what you've tried isn't working and you need another perspective. You've shared enough of yourself that they can see how to help, and they *want* to help. Let them. Remember that people can move in and out of your village, so redo this assessment from time to time so you know where to focus your energy.

One key piece of information to be mindful of is that once you have unpotted and transplanted yourself into a more nourishing environment, you will not be able to go back to the old environment. Think about our tomato plant. After moving it into a larger container, its root structure stretches out, digging through the wider expanse of soil it has been given access to. What we see above the soil is also larger and stronger. If we attempt to pull it out of the larger container and put it back in the starter container, it simply will not fit. It can't. It's outgrown that way of life.

When you transplant yourself into a space that fosters your growth, gives you opportunities to change how you think, and feeds your soul, you will have outgrown the old space. Trying to repot yourself after you've been transplanted is like trying to ooze back into last summer's skinny jeans, having devoured the mountain of unsold Girl Scout cookies left over after a brutal season. Part of the unpotting process is releasing the old space, the old way of life, and acknowledging that it is no longer for you.

This contributes to the discomfort because we like what is familiar. We like knowing what is expected. We like having backup plans. Backup plans are fine, and they need to be focused on forward momentum, not falling back to places we've outgrown.

Don't worry, you were made for this. You've got this, and your village has you. This is a hard thing. You can do hard things, and you can do them incredibly well. You already are - you've taken your first steps into the Soul Alchemy Cycle. You're building the muscles you will need to help yourself find the healing you so deeply deserve.

4

THE B WORD

What even is burnout, anyway? The word is used so ubiquitously in current culture that it seems like it can be applied to anything and everything related to a bit of stress. It's mostly used about work, but not exclusively. I know several people who have discussed friendships that have burned them out, or being burned out on hobbies.

Burnout is a word that has become almost a non-word, applied with only a modicum of understanding its meaning. It could describe the deep feeling of detachment from things you once enjoyed to the point of dread. It could also describe temporary boredom or overwhelm that will dissipate with a week or two break.

In this book, I focus on that first, more penetrating definition of burnout. I'm examining the phenomenon that happens when a person is broken by something they were once empowered by. There is a massive industry that has been built up around addressing this form and helping people recover. I spent a fair amount of time working through what that industry had to offer because I was desperate to find passion and power in my work again. Some of it would work for a little while, but over and over, I would relapse into the malignant disconnection and despair that exemplified my post-response existence.

The challenges I experienced in managing my own burnout and using resources from this massive industry came down to the fact that the resources were too superficial in their approach. In order to come up with a method that would dig out the issue at the source, I needed to understand what the industry was basing its approach on. I could build on that knowledge to find a way to stop relapsing. Healing was my goal, not treatment. Bandage solutions weren't the path for me, and I'm guessing they're not for you either.

A Brief History Lesson

Burnout, as we culturally know it, was first described in the mid-1970s by two psychologists working independently. Herbert Freudenberger and Christina Maslach both studied people working in the service sector, including medical professionals, firefighters, police, and clergy. They noticed patterns of behavior in these workers after exposure to extreme and/or prolonged stress. Overwork, idealism, exhaustion, anger, and over-commitment were widely present in these populations.

Freudenberger coined the term 'burnout' as a proxy for these symptoms under one umbrella, borrowing it from the drug scene as he was working at a free substance abuse clinic in New York at the time. Maslach collaborated with Susan E Jackson to develop a framework for understanding and quantifying burnout in an individual.

Maslach's framework, the original Maslach Burnout Inventory, looks at three dimensions of burnout, including emotional exhaustion, depersonalization, and personal accomplishment. This framework has been enhanced by developing five new versions to focus on different occupational groups and settings. These new versions also measure cynicism and professional efficacy.

Big Structures, Small Solutions

The tools and understanding brought by Freudenberger, Maslach, and Jackson have been instrumental in treating innumerable individuals with burnout and getting them back to a manageable level of productivity while reducing their stress levels. However, this model places all of the burden of managing burnout, all of the responsibility for it happening in the first place, on the individual experiencing it.

If you don't understand the underlying cause, you'll only ever be treating symptoms.

Current wisdom is dedicated to treating symptoms and providing supportive care until someone is able to get back to their expected baseline. The model doesn't examine the underlying cause. If you don't understand the underlying cause, you'll only ever be treating symptoms.

At its root, burnout is caused and supported by systemic structures and cultural expectations. The social contracts we have developed around what is expected of each of us as individuals reinforce the environment where burnout is allowed to exist. When this environment is not addressed, people who have experienced burnout relapse, and more people fall into the pit of burnout.

Supportive care absolutely has a place. It is the best option when there is no reasonable way to address the underlying cause. We see this when someone contracts a virus that doesn't have an antiviral developed. There's no tool to address the virus, so we focus on supporting the patient's body so their immune system can take care of the virus naturally.

Addressing systemic structures, cultural expectations, and social contracts is big. Too big. We haven't developed a tool to do this yet without throwing all of society into complete upheaval. The default, then, becomes supportive care for those who are experiencing symptoms. The solution is a bandage, and we have to hope that the patient's mental equivalent of an immune system is strong enough to weather the storm.

This defeatist attitude doesn't sit well with me, not least because I've discovered a way to address the root cause on an individual level. I'm not trying to change all of society. I'm simply choosing to change how I interact with it. I'm making a conscious decision not to buy into the social contracts driving this phenomenon while simultaneously living and working among those who continue to. Being able to do this requires a lot of mental exercise, beginning with understanding the myths those social contracts are built on. So buckle up, we're going on a ride.

Ugly Foundations

The culture we live in is so deeply dependent on productivity that society as we know it cannot be sustained without it. We saw in 2020 how, near globally, there was a collective rush to get back to 'normal' and get people back into their workplaces prematurely. When that didn't work, companies embraced remote work to the point where remote working became a basic expectation of employees.

Those that couldn't produce through remote work were declared essential, whether they actually played a role in ensuring necessities of living were properly distributed or not. Workers in restaurants, for instance, were told to choose between coming back in person and working or being unemployed – and this was before masking was widely adopted. There was total disregard for the individual and their health, so long as the company survived.

Certainly, not every business operated this way, and enough to make it an observable trend did. At the surface level, this makes sense. A company has bills to pay whether they are open or not, whether they are generating revenue or not. Most businesses don't have enough reserves to weather a long closure, so they have to come up with ways to survive. That frequently involves making tough choices and rarely works out in favor of the individual employees.

On a societal level, this continued to play out over the following years as well. More and more people were wishing the pandemic to be over so strongly that they simply decided it was over, beginning to behave in such a way that facilitated spread and mutation. As company leaders adopted this head-in-the-sand stance, those under them were left with little choice but to follow – or risk losing their own livelihood.

These attitudes spread almost as virulently as the disease itself and carried with them a disregard for those who couldn't keep up. The people most at risk of serious complications or death from contracting COVID-19, those with comorbidities that produced disability, were left behind as the attitude of returning to 'normalcy' prevailed.

This demographic had the burden of maintaining all of the precautions that had been in place during the pandemic, but at an enhanced level, both because of their physical health and because nobody else was contributing to a precautionary environment. This societal decision to dump the burden of caution on the people who had the fewest resources to implement and maintain it exemplified the view that this group of human beings was disposable. They couldn't produce, so society couldn't be bothered to consider them.

This is not a bug. This is a feature of how our culture is currently structured. Shifting responsibility for mitigating the impacts of societal failings to the individual who is least prepared to handle them is a habit we see playing out over and over.

It shows up in how we currently treat burnout, too. Not only is the whole goal of the existing supportive care model to get you back to work and producing, it is you, the burned out individual, who must make that happen with tools inadequate for the job.

Just stress less. Make sure you get back to producing more. It's in your hands. Why can't you stop stressing? Why aren't you producing? What's wrong with you? If you followed this more closely, more rigorously, you wouldn't have so much stress. Maybe try this other method or this other book or podcast. Have you tried yoga?

Someone asked me why my ideas on how to heal burnout are different from the current methods, in that both require the burned out person to be in the driver's seat. That's a fair question because it's true. You are the one who has to figure out your specific situation and how to get out of it.

You are the one who knows you best, and so I firmly believe that you are the one who should be in charge of your recovery. Being in charge doesn't mean being unsupported, though. It also doesn't mean being blamed.

The difference is in culpability. Rugged individualism, a key feature of our culture, insists that if you can't do something, it's your fault. If you can't fix yourself, only you are to blame. And this situation you find yourself in? Well, if you'd been a little tougher, you wouldn't be here in the first place.

I'm here to tell you it's not always your fault. Do you screw up sometimes? Sure, so do I. We're human, and we make mistakes. Not everything that goes wrong in life is your fault, though. Sometimes, it's a matter of being enmeshed in patterns that started long before your existence was contemplated.

And you have the power to break those patterns.

Exercise 3: Releasing the Burden

Spend a little extra time on this exercise. This is some big unpotting work because you're going to be challenging some deep-seated beliefs about your world, so tap into your gardening tools as you begin.

Name three things that you feel responsible for fixing. For each thing you have listed, work through the following questions.

🍃 Why do you feel responsible for fixing this?

🍃 Is it something that keeps you up at night or distracts you from your work?

🍃 Are you blaming yourself for this situation existing in the first place?

  🍃 If so, what does the voice say to you when you blame yourself?

  🍃 Is it true?

  🍃 Whose voice is it? Is it actually yours, or is it someone else's that you've internalized?

🍃 What power does this thing hold over you?

  🍃 Who or what gave it that power?

  🍃 Is it valid?

After you have completed assessing all three things on your list with these questions, ask yourself which burdens can be released. Which are yours, and which belong elsewhere? Your responsibility is absolutely to take action from here forward, and you don't need to be carrying responsibility that isn't yours. Place it on the ground and walk away with your head held high.

Challenging enmeshed patterns is some big work, and you're doing it! There's another enmeshed pattern living in your head that you might not realize is there - or how heavy it is. Big breaths here, we're going to go right up against the granddaddy of them all: your productivity as a measure of your personal worth.

The Myth of Productivity

Productivity is king in our culture, and those who produce a lot are venerated and held up as a shining beacon that all should aspire to. Those who are unable to produce are considered worthless, burdensome, contemptible. It wasn't that long ago that our society decided hiding our non-producers in institutions with minimal oversight was maybe not such a good look.

The attitudes that locked those people up for the crime of existing as themselves still fester.

You and I have been steeped in this culture to prove we are good little producers, worthy of being an active part of society since we put on backpacks that overshadowed our tiny statures and walked across the school threshold for the first time. The easiest example of how this concept was introduced to us was through extra credit – do more work, get a better grade. Working a bit harder in class is likely to earn regard from the teacher, which comes in awful handy when you need a bit of leniency on something.

If you don't do your homework, though, regardless of the reason, you could easily end up in detention. It doesn't matter if the concept was one you couldn't quite grasp without more help or if you had responsibilities at home that ate up all of your time. Not producing is punished; producing is rewarded. We learn this young, and it follows us into adulthood.

We learn to segregate one another into productive or not productive, worthy or unworthy. We quickly hone the skill of placing someone along that spectrum as we grow, guiding us in our decisions about how much

67

we should interact with one another. As children, we can't even recognize that we are buying into this social contract. We accept it without knowing there is a choice to be had. Our friend groups, study groups, and role models are decided for us based on this spectrum.

We acknowledge that someone can move up or down on that spectrum based on individual effort, and we romanticize people who increase their standing 'against all odds' and through significant personal turmoil. We indulge in inspiration porn and use it as evidence that we, too, can make something of ourselves if we just work harder. When we don't end up actually changing our circumstances, we take it as a personal failure instead of objectively assessing the situation.

That finish line is forever shifting. You will never cross it because you're not meant to.

If that one person who defied the odds could work their way up from so much further down the socio-economic ladder than I'm at, why can't I just get a little bit further ahead? What are they doing that I'm not? What's wrong with me?

Reviewing the situation as an observer rather than someone actively involved in it, you may notice that the requirements of success keep changing. The goal is never the same. Once you reach a certain goal, that's great but no longer enough to be considered above average. Getting a little further ahead just means barely keeping up. It's not enough to gain regard, to gain worthiness of extra resources. What can you do now? And now? And now?

That finish line is forever shifting. You will never cross it because you're not meant to. If you crossed it, there would be no incentive for you to produce more, and our culture insists on productivity from every human in it.

You can't hold onto the myth of productivity and avoid burnout. You have to release it to create space for your new understanding of yourself and the world around you.

Exercise 4: Letting Go

Back in Chapter 1, I asked you to imagine what you would do with your time absent any obligations or financial barriers. We didn't do a full-fledged exercise about it then; they were just questions to ponder. We're going to do one now that you have more information on how this insipid myth that has been part of your social landscape your entire life impacts your answers.

Set a timer for 15 minutes for this exercise. Answer instinctively; don't overthink your response. Remember that there are no right or wrong answers in these exercises. This is about you, where you're at, and where you're moving toward.

As you progress through the following questions, note first what your answer was when you read through the prompts in Chapter 1. Then, review the prompt again through the lens of releasing the idea that you must always be productive.

🍃 How would you spend your time if you had no obligations and money was no object?

🍃 How would your day flow in this world you've built?

 🍃 Your week?

 🍃 Your year?

🍃 Is your instinct to plan things to accomplish or ways of existing? Why?

 🍃 If it's a mix of the two, which is weighted more heavily? Why?

🍃 Would your answer bring you to a place of peace and contentment?

🍃 Would you regret your answer after living in it for a year?

 🍃 Five years?

 🍃 Ten years?

Did your answers change? What emotions went through you as you looked at these questions from a new perspective? Even the smallest shift in your answers here means you are well on your way to releasing the myth of productivity and stepping into your new world - a world where you alone define your worth.

Pricing Out the Unproductive

Our culture needs us to continuously produce so very much that it has forged infrastructure intended to enshrine this myth of productivity in our socioeconomic consciousness. The majority of people in this culture are steeped in a scarcity mindset by having a price attributed to our specific kind and level of productivity. That price drives our access to basic needs, like shelter, food, safety, healthcare, and utility services. It also impacts the quality of what is available to us in each of those categories and so many more.

This infrastructure is the perfect place to hide abuses of power. Classes of people with immutable characteristics can have their efforts priced differently, and there is a nominally plausible (read: not plausible at all, but it makes those in power feel better about themselves) reason that can be given as to why they deserve less. Perhaps they don't have as much education or experience as others, or maybe they are physically not capable of producing as much because of a disability. These proxy reasons, though, are a feature of the infrastructure and are self-fulfilling.

When a person in this situation is paid less for their efforts, they do not have the same opportunity to support their basic needs and further their education – or that of their children. They don't have the means to support their children through unpaid internships, providing experience that can be leveraged to launch their careers. They do not have the ability to take time off of work and focus on rest that nourishes their bodies and minds. These people are easy to take advantage of because they are scrambling to simply survive; they do not have the privilege of fighting back against abusive workplaces.

The P Word

So, what exactly is privilege? Look back to Chapter 1 for a basic definition, and then let's talk here about it a bit more. Contrary to what many would have you believe, it's not something that automatically shields your life from pain. You can hold privilege and still work through significant challenges. Privileges do, however, make the way easier. People with less privilege have to do twice as much to be seen as half as worthy as those who hold many privileges.

Privilege acts like a suit of armor. Imagine with me, for a moment, you are a medieval knight with a forest in front of you that you must traverse to reach home. The more pieces of that armor you wear on your travels, the fewer perils in your path you will notice, much less be impacted by. Sabatons and greaves protect the lower legs and feet, so it's doubtful you'd be aware of walking through a bed of thistle on the forest edge that might otherwise snag, poke, and tangle your legs.

You'd still notice bumping into a thick branch poking out from some brush, but it would be an annoyance easily ignored rather than something that did damage to your leg or slowed you down. Add in some knee cops, cuisses for your upper legs, and a cuirass for your torso, and you can handle most things coming your way with ease. Top it off with a helmet, and that falling branch will be a headache rather than a journey-ending event.

Why the heck am I going on about all of this? You picked up a book about how to fix your burnout, not to get a lecture on social issues, and certainly not to learn about medieval armor. Right now, it feels like we are so far off topic that we won't ever get back. Stick with me here – the lightbulb moment is just around the corner.

All of this is crucial context for understanding the root cause of burnout. The systemic structures, cultural expectations, and social contracts we just touched on – very lightly, mind you – are the foundation of why you are burned out. Built on this foundation is the professional culture we operate in. It's the polite, polished face of the productivity myth, privilege, and hidden abuses.

Office Spaces

Professional culture demands conformity: conformity of thought, conformity of behavior, and conformity of appearance. Behind conformity is the idea that there is an Ideal Person who is the most productive member of society, and the more we try to emulate that person in every way, the more productive we will be seen as. Our Ideal Person checks all the boxes of privilege, and the more we produce, the closer we can get to holding those privileges ourselves. Those who start out with a full suit of privilege armor don't have nearly as far to go.

Management philosophies enforce this conformity to try to enhance productivity within their work unit. A manager's role, regardless of the level, company, or sector, is to inspire those they manage to ever-increasing levels of productivity. It's how a manager produces. This can lead to environments where management says one thing to their workers to increase engagement while never planning on acting on it because it would take resources away from producing more. Change isn't the goal here; production is.

These environments then foster a culture of not seeing the human doing the work and not supporting the needs of that human. Have you ever been in a place where you completed work ahead of schedule and above and beyond expectations? If so, I would bet good money that you were rewarded for that work with a pile of more work. If you received some kind of acknowledgement for your efforts other than more work, was it meaningful? Or was it a trinket like a pen or a mug with the company's logo, or – worse –

a form letter with the signature printed rather than signed in actual ink?

Perfunctory, mass-produced recognition doesn't meet our human need to be seen. Neither does a load of new work, even if it's couched as being given a higher level of responsibility. It's a classic tactic of professional culture to dangle these trifles in front of us with the implicit promise that if we work a bit harder, produce a bit more, we'll receive the recognition and support that we need and deserve.

You have been taught that chasing an illusion was the only way to be seen for who you are.

The problem is, that carrot doesn't exist. The ideal person is perfect, and perfect isn't real. You've been sweet talked to your whole life about how to finally, finally be recognized for the amazing human you are. You've denied yourself happiness in pursuit of a mirage more than once. You've turned yourself into a machine whose only goal is to produce because you were assured that was the way to have your needs met.

That right there is the deep, true, full root cause of your burnout: you have been taught that chasing an illusion was the only way to be seen for who you are. It's time to step off the merry-go-round of productivity and embrace that you are a human being. You are *not* a human doing. You deserve happiness, rest, and freedom.

Walk with me a little further, and I'll show you the way.

albedo

purify

5

GRAMMAR'S COOL

A fresh crop of new colleagues sat with me around a utilitarian table, one of those made from particle board and covered in a veneer of faux-granite vinyl, that took up the majority of the tiny conference room we had been able to secure. The sun hovered over the lake just outside our building, creating a double glare that blinded anyone foolish enough to glance at the singular window illuminating this space. It was their first day, and it was the second time I had run the four-week orientation program I had designed for my work unit, which audited Medicaid claims.

Some of them sat very rigidly in their rolling chairs while others tapped pens nervously or paged through the binders in front of them. Each was a Registered

Nurse, and several looked uncomfortable in business casual rather than their broken-in scrubs.

I cleared my throat and dove into the day's business. My first question startled all of them out of their assumed postures and threw them off guard a little bit: "Why did you take this job?" Answers ranged from rote interview answers of "looking for a challenge" or "wanting to explore a new area of nursing practice" to a much blunter "I was tired of working weekends and holidays." All are valid reasons, and none were quite what I was asking.

After we went around the table, I shared my reason. Medicaid saved my life and the lives of my children by providing access to top-quality providers and facilities, and I wanted to give back to the program that gave so much to my family. One person spoke up and said, "Well, that was much deeper than any of ours."

I smiled.

After three years in the role, I'd had much more time to think about my answer than these folks had, and I shared with them that was a large part of the point. I encouraged them to spend some time over the following several weeks of orientation thinking about their *why*, not just on the surface but at a more intuitive level. Auditing definitely had some interesting moments, and 80% of it was repetitive, monotonous work. It's a very different environment and way of working from clinical practice, where most of my new colleagues had come from.

Without a strong *why*, it would be very easy for them to lose focus on our larger mission while buried in the daily minutiae and decrease their satisfaction in their work. A *why* was critical. It provided an anchor when they got frustrated, a lighthouse to guide them when they felt lost, and comfort when they felt discouraged.

Defining Purpose

Developing and shepherding this exercise was the first step into my understanding the word *purpose* differently. Just about every definition I can find for purpose denotes it as a noun. It's a reason for existing, an end, aim, or goal. The English language comfortably transmutes this word to fit a multitude of contexts, and they almost exclusively mean something to be achieved. Purpose is a *what* in all of these definitions.

In this sense, purpose is very heavily tied to productivity and to measures of worth. A person must reach their goal in order to have fulfilled their purpose. When a thing stops working after performing a task repeatedly over a period of time, it is said that it has served its purpose. A purpose is a destination. It is something to be reached and completed. Its existence is temporary. After it is done, a new purpose must be found in order for the item or person to continue to have worth.

Each of us is constantly looking for our next what, convinced that this will be the one that finally brings us what we need.

Think back to Chapter 4 and how this definition feeds into the productivity myth that drives burnout. It feeds the cycle of working toward a nonexistent reward because once the task is done – once the purpose is fulfilled – what can you do for me now? Each of us is constantly looking for our next *what*, convinced that this will be the one that finally brings us what we need. Our pursuit of success, happiness, or whatever word you want to substitute there always comes back to looking for the next *what.*

My shift into the pandemic response in May of 2020 was a really good *what.* It felt good for a long time. I was filled with this old version of purpose, a noun with an end goal. My team's goal was to contain a virus and support our population while we were doing it. I internalized that proto-purpose.

As it became more obvious that we would never contain the virus, I switched my focus to creating sustainable supportive IT infrastructure for the next emergency. I had a new proto-purpose, one that warranted a permanent role doing this work. I remember the feeling with each move, *this is the one that will change everything. This is the one that will convince people of my worth for good.*

Of course, it wasn't. It never would be. A big part of that is that I was still thinking about purpose in completely the wrong context.

Purpose as an Adjective

Purpose, as I use it in this book and in my daily life, is an adjective. It doesn't tell you what I'm seeking to accomplish; rather, it describes me. My purpose describes the core nature of myself. It doesn't end while I still exist. There is no next what to look for with this definition. When I began to ask myself, "what is your why?" in relation to my life rather than only for my work, I started defining my personal purpose. I clarified who I was, how I would make decisions, and what was most important to the core me absent any of my obligations.

Once your purpose is defined and you actively begin to describe yourself in terms of a purpose statement, you build a framework for how you move through the world. When a choice is presented to you, you have the ability to step back and assess your situation. Is this particular issue in line with your purpose? Is it in harmony with how you describe yourself?

If so, proceed joyfully. If not, examine more closely why it is drawing your attention in the first place. The clarity received from shining the light of your purpose on your actions or potential actions gives you the confidence to move forward without hesitation.

When I look back at my decision to move into the pandemic response and compare it to my defined purpose, it is in full alignment. That's why I think it felt good for such a long time. Not only was I filled with the old version of purpose, the move aligned with my purpose-as-an-adjective, though I didn't understand the concept at that point.

The subsequent shifts could have benefitted from being held up against the light of my purpose-as-an-adjective. I may have chosen differently and not become run down as much, but I didn't have that tool to provide clarity when I was making those choices.

I won't lie; simply holding your purpose and knowing your *why* does not guarantee smooth sailing. There will always be barriers to break through, mountains to climb, and moments of friction in life that have you asking, "Why am I doing this?" The good news, though, is that you have that *why* to wield as an anchor, an inextinguishable lantern to illuminate your journey, and the warmest, softest blanket to wrap around yourself in comfort. It is a multifaceted tool and the most powerful one you own.

This is the primary reason I included the exercise at the beginning of the onboarding process. Without a *why*, I knew my new colleagues would lose focus on the bigger picture. Without your purpose-as-an-adjective, it can be easy to lose hope when life gets tough, even when something is exactly what you are supposed to be doing.

When you hit the barriers life throws your way and ask yourself why you are doing the thing, take a moment to hold the thing up to your purpose. Is it in alignment with your why? If yes, remind yourself of all of the ways it is connected to how you describe yourself. Go into detail; this will reconnect you to the meaning behind the thing and provide you with the courage to move through the rough time, knowing that continuing the work is a worthwhile use of your resources.

If not, pay attention. That's exactly where you are going to find yourself falling into burnout over and over again.

You may be thinking, "This sounds great! What's my purpose? How do I figure it out? When do we start?" Believe it or not, you've already started. Recognizing that you need to define this purpose-as-an-adjective means your roots have reached the limits of your growing container, and you're ready to start unpotting yourself. Remember that repotting is uncomfortable, so plan how you will nourish yourself as you wade into the journey.

6

WHAT VS. WHY

I was a very curious child. It drove my mother nuts. When I wasn't asking her a series of incessant 'why' questions about random things, I was busy poking my fingers in places they didn't belong. I wanted to understand the world around me, not only the objects and what they did, but why they worked the way they did and why they were necessary in the first place. This curiosity and the energy behind it earned me the nickname of Busy Fingers at a young age.

At age six, I decided I would be an inventor when I grew up. I had so many ideas rattling around inside my head and I wanted to bring them into reality because they were, to my thinking, really good ideas. I would grab items from around the house and tie or tape them together to try to make something else. As those things go, some worked better than others. The others resulted in various degrees of hilarious catastrophe. I got really good at cleaning.

I'd learn, though, that each idea I had was something that someone else had already thought of and was an existing product that could be bought. Instead of taking away the lesson that I was on the right track in questioning the world around me and developing new ways to do things, I learned that my ideas were unoriginal and not worth pursuing.

I learned to stuff my curiosity and creativity into the back corner of my mind to keep my Busy Fingers tied up and pursue more traditional ways of contributing to society. Ways like accounting (I legitimately wanted to be a CPA when I was 12) or medicine (ages 14-18, and again at 27). My father would brag to colleagues about the things I wanted to be and how I, his daughter, would contribute to society. I learned how to focus on a *what* – a thing to do, a goal to attain – rather than questioning and looking for *whys*.

More, I learned that finding a *what* defined my personal worth, and that worth shifted significantly depending on which *what* I chose. Those lessons were reinforced through young adulthood as I struggled through the bottom of the career ecosystem. In social settings, I'd frequently find ways to disguise or fluff up what I did for a living. If I shared my job title as my employer defined it, I would be deemed less interesting to talk to or invest time and energy in.

It didn't matter that, as an administrative assistant, I kept an office running and ensured several people had what they needed to produce at a higher level. Their work – their *what* – literally produced something, so they were more valuable, more worthy than me.

It wasn't just familial pressures at this point anymore; there was a cultural push, a drive, to produce as much as possible, as fast as possible. Only then would I be deemed worthy of the resources and energy necessary to keep me alive, to support my family, to live a comfortable life. I had fully bought into the myth that productivity was the sole answer to success, and that if I tried hard enough, I could actually pull myself up by my bootstraps and be successful.

The thing about bootstraps, though, is that if you manage to physically pull them up, against gravity and your own mass, your feet are off the ground. You can't stand. You tip over and fall face first into the dirt. It's impossible to actually accomplish, and the laws of physics don't care about how determined you are. The Bootstraps Myth is another myth our culture is built on; it's the sibling myth to the Productivity Myth we covered in Chapter 4.

These two myths did an excellent job of putting my desire for a why on a high shelf in a dusty corner and blocking it with a tangled clutter of emotions: guilt, with its jagged edges biting into the wood of the shelf to make sure it stayed firmly in place; fear, a bulky, moth-eaten blanket, jumbled up in a ball rather than folded neatly; sadness, a child's 3rd grade science project gone half-wrong, broken and limp but holding too much attachment to actually dispose of. Ugly, painful emotions not fit for public consumption that are best kept hidden.

After all, the what would lead to success as I knew it.

Disrupting them, even a gentle poke or tug, was so painful and consumed so much energy that I abandoned attempts at cleaning out the corner shelf.

I had no energy left after devoting my whole self into fostering my *what*. After all, the *what* would lead to success as I knew it. Curiosity and creativity had no place in that pursuit, so it was a better, safer, more practical choice to allot my resources toward being as productive as possible. I could earn my worth, and everyone would see it because I'd be rewarded with status and luxury.

You already know where that definition of success landed me. Allowing someone else – some nameless, nebulous person or persons – to prescribe exactly what my life should look like, what I should aspire to, how I should be rewarded or chastised left me pursuing a mirage. It was an oasis in an endless desert that I could see but never reach, ever shifting further away as I clawed my exhausted body across the sharp grains of sand, desperate for a drop of water on my lips.

Most people will live the rest of their lives this way. It's all they know. There is not another way in their minds because they have not been shown another way. They haven't been taught to be curious, to question the world around them or how it works. Their natural instinct was shut down at a very young age and tucked up high on a shelf behind a bevy of dusty, ugly emotions.

Some have even walled off that corner with the bricks labeled 'discipline.' They will stay in this uncurious, unquestioning place to their last breath because the pain of staying the same never exceeds the pain of tearing down the wall and pulling away the emotions. They are not willing to get uncomfortable.

That's not how we operate around here, though. We intentionally get uncomfortable - we unpot ourselves on the regular - and we do hard things! Let's do one of those now and dig into your own dusty corner.

Exercise 5: Spring Cleaning

Grab your favorite documenting tools, find a comfortable spot, and spend about 20 minutes going through these prompts. Respond instinctively; don't spend too long thinking about your answers.

❀ What did you want to be when you grew up at age:

    ❀ 5?

    ❀ 9?

    ❀ 14?

    ❀ 18?

    ❀ 25?

❀ What influenced the changes between each age?

    ❀ Were you introduced to new ideas?

    ❀ Did you feel pressure to move away from something? If so, what kind?

        ❀ Where did that pressure come from?

        ❀ What pressures were most influential?

❀ If you could choose anything to do now, without restriction on money/time/education (assume you have plenty of all of them for the rest of your life), what would you do?

- 🌿 Is your choice creative or productive?

- 🌿 Why do you lean the way you do?

- 🌿 Does thinking about this bring up any emotions? If so, what kinds?

- 🌿 Where and when did you first start feeling those emotions around how you move through the world?

After finishing this exercise, review your answers and sit with them for a moment. What parts of them are based in reality? What have you been told that keeps you focused on a *what* rather than leaning into your *why*?

The Real Oasis

The pain of leaning into a *what* had brought me to my knees, and I knew I couldn't continue living in that agony. Even more than my own pain, though, I worried about what my example would do to my children. Was I dooming them to a lifetime of chasing mirages, always dissatisfied, just because I wasn't willing to do the work of cleaning out my dusty corner?

They saw me reach a modicum of social success. They watched me crawl from the bottom of the career ecosystem to somewhere in the middle, with moderate rewards that looked pretty good compared to what we'd previously lived with. I'd already put myself through so much to ensure they had good childhoods. I decided that I could endure the pain of change again and figure all of this out for their sake.

I enlisted the help of a wonderful therapist to start pulling those painful emotions down, not knowing that's what I was doing at the time. During our first meeting, I told her one of my main goals of therapy was to figure out what was getting in the way of my success. What was preventing me from moving further up in the career ecosystem? My mind still defined success in terms of productivity: what exactly was wrong with my *what*, and how do I fix it? More precisely, what was wrong with *me*?

Over the course of our work, we pulled the guilt, fear, and sadness around my creative self out of that dusty corner, examined them, and processed them.

101

Simply getting them down allowed me a glimpse of that creativity box; I could peek in the corner of the lid and ask why again. Curiosity came back. I started having more trust in my ideas and more willingness to share them with those around me.

It didn't take long for my questions to aim themselves at the world I'd created around me and the decisions I made. This curiosity and willingness to question myself without judgment primed me to delve the depths of my core self and discover my purpose. I could finally ask why about myself. Not why do I do a thing, but why am I? Why am I here, in this place, at this time? Why do I matter?

This was my first step into moving through what is now the Soul Alchemy Cycle: asking why about myself, over and over, until I found the root answer. My purpose-as-an-adjective. This asking required me to deconstruct what I thought I knew about the world. It forced me to assess my drive for productivity and why I couldn't let go of it. It insisted I let that fade away. It demanded I examine why I permitted a nebulous other to define what my success looked like. It permitted me to see how I could be the master of my own success, not subject to the whims of others.

As it turns out, that curiosity I was born with and wielded so naturally as a child is an incredibly powerful tool. Asking why brings up uncomfortable answers for those who wish to maintain the status quo. It's easier to stifle those questions, that curiosity, and lock it away behind pain than it is to risk answering honestly.

Having the courage to rip through that pain, to let it wash over you, understand it, and release it gives you access to your innate power. It gives you the freedom to begin to understand yourself. It allows you to watch your *what* melt into oblivion to make room for your fiercely growing *why*.

citrinitas

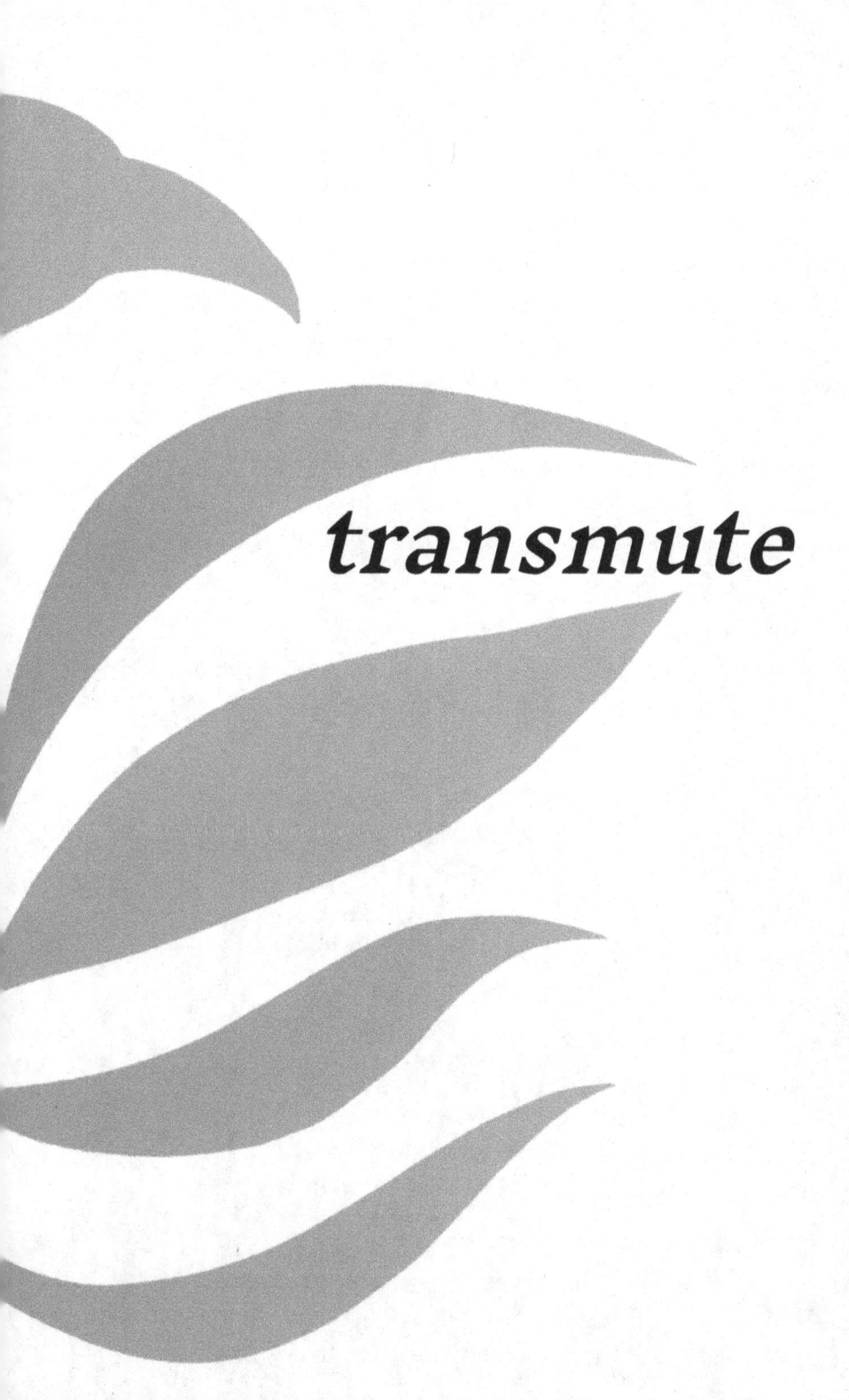

transmute

7

FINDING YOURSELF

One random Tuesday morning, my traditional forgotten cold coffee in hand, I was helping a friend work through this process. She said something in our discussion that made me put my coffee down and forget it some more. She told me that she had to include her children and nominally estranged husband among the people who were important to her.

I asked her to stop before we went any further and feel through the word 'had' and what it meant for her situation. Basically, she felt obligated to include these people in her list because, societally, if she didn't, she would be viewed as a bad mother and wife. Those identities that were pushing themselves to the forefront in this conversation were part of a societal norm; they were learned, not innate.

Learned identities are something you and I were socialized into, starting when we could begin to communicate. First, we are someone's child. Then, we are someone's friend. Then, a student. A partner. An employee. A citizen. A parent. There are so many other identities we take on as we grow through life, and each one carries its own set of norms and requirements for masking who we are. We code-switch as we navigate these identities, and when two or more identities collide, we think nothing of allowing the strictest one to take precedence.

What if you prioritized your obligation to yourself first?

The vast majority of our learned identities are who we are in relation to other people. Our obligations are to those people. We put their needs first to ensure we are fulfilling society's norms. We sacrifice our own needs to ensure theirs are met first.

What if you prioritized your obligation to yourself first? You might find that your core self breathes a sigh of relief, finally able to put down the heavy weight of your pile of learned identities. The irritations that chafe inside your mind as you perform those identities melt away into nothing. Many authorities in the mental health space call this practice setting and maintaining boundaries. Whatever you choose to call it, it comes down to the same thing – your core self's needs must be met before you have the capacity to give to others.

So, who exactly is your core self, and what do you need? How do you strip away all of these learned identities to discover that core self?

Simply put, your core self is the essence of who you are. It may be shaped by relationships and experiences much the same way a potter shapes a lump of clay, but your core self is the lump of clay, not the mug or vase that someone else influences into form. It is composed of your individual values, your emotions, your hopes, and your dreams. We'll delve into meeting your core self's needs in Chapters 9 and 10, after you've had a chance to dig deep and name that self.

Planting Seeds

In November of 2021, I was at my most broken to date. It was then that Dr. Jasmine Zapata came to our Division's all-staff meeting and spoke of purpose. She shared the purpose board that she had developed; it was similar to a vision board, but instead of including goals and dreams, the purpose board included visual reminders of who she was and why she did what she did.

I was so excited about this idea of having an individual purpose and making a purpose board that I brought it to a network I was a part of and shared it. If I found it useful, someone else might too, right? I figured I'd pass it on and be done with it.

Of course, life had other plans. The idea was so well received that the moderators asked if I'd be willing to lead a class on it. My inability to say no leaped to the forefront, and I blurted out an enthusiastic "yes!" before the rest of my brain had actually processed what was happening.

I am so grateful for the gentle, gracious black woman who was the catalyst of everything that happened in that network. It was only with her continuous nudging that I was able to put together the puzzle pieces of the base process for discerning one's purpose so that I could teach it to a group. I'm a thorough researcher, so I put myself through the paces of what I would be teaching and stumbled face-first into this need to strip away my learned identities.

Peeling Back the Layers

Stripping your learned identities from your core self is not an easy task. Like many worthwhile things, it takes time and practice to learn and a lifetime to master. You have lived for so long with each of these identities that they feel very much like the core of you.

I challenge you, the same way I challenged my friend, to *shed the should*. As you work through the exercises in this chapter and the next, any time the words 'should' or 'have to' come up in your explanation of why someone or something needs to be included, pause and question it.

Ask yourself, what exactly is your obligation? Is it an obligation to another person? Is the obligation to society or its norms? Is the obligation to yourself?

Be critical of the answer and really feel it out. The answer shouldn't come easily; like you, each decision is built of many facets. If it does, you likely need to sit with it and examine it more.

When you've finished examining your answer, if the obligation is connected to any learned identity, consider leaving it out. You don't need to apply this questioning process for every single item that comes up in these exercises. Keep it only for when you feel the tug of obligation rather than certainty and ease.

Once you have begun to remove those learned identities, it's time to start investigating who you are as a human. This part is easier, and I invite you to be conscious of your learned identities trying to creep into it. Even though this process was much easier, keeping those learned identities at bay was absolutely the hardest part for me as I walked this journey. It was so easy to slip into mom-me or employee-me.

You already know so much about those identities. You live them every day in every way. You're trying to discover your core self; make sure that core self has space to speak.

The Pieces of You

There are five key components to explore when walking this journey. You'll spend quite a bit of time focusing on these components in the exercises in this chapter and Chapter 8, so slow down and become familiar with each and what they entail before you proceed.

Personal Artifacts

"What is this," you might be thinking, "an archaeological dig?" Well, kind of. Instead of studying an historical culture, though, you are studying historical you. Personal artifacts are those things we carry with us through life, no matter what.

They may be in a box in storage that you open once a decade (if that) to remember people or events. They may be something you proudly display in your home so they can help establish the energy of your home. You cannot bring yourself to get rid of these items, even if they break. If your home burned down, losing them would break your heart.

Things that Bring You Joy

Without a doubt, some of your personal artifacts will bring you joy. However, this component looks at more mundane things. These could be physical items or experiences. The big one that jumped out for me was lipstick. There are few things in the world that make me happier than a really good lipstick formula in a color I can rock.

Another sampling from my journey is an experience. I have a tradition between Thanksgiving and Christmas after the tree is set up and sparkling with the eclectic assortment of ornaments that exemplifies my family's chaotic and glorious way of being.

I will get up very early, before anyone else is up and while the house is quiet, and get myself something warm and soothing to drink (usually coffee that ends up going cold in my hands, but what can you do?). Then, I'll put on some soft instrumental Christmas music, curl up under a blanket with only the lights of the tree on, and bask in its ethereal beauty. I've had this tradition since I was 7 or 8, and I hope to continue it as long as I'm alive. It is my happy place.

Things that Bring You Pride

A quick note here – pride in and of itself has no morality to it. It's ok to be proud of something. It's ok to celebrate that pride. So, what makes you want to puff your chest out and tell the world about it? What makes you wish town criers were still a thing so they could shout out your news to everyone around you? What makes you run to your favorite social media platform to gleefully share with all of your contacts since that's the closest thing to a town crier that exists right now?

My top entry here is when I complete a challenging task that had been baffling me. Nothing makes me prouder than looking at something hard, getting into the muck of it, questioning whether I can actually do it, and then pushing my way across the finish line anyway. What fills your soul that way?

Things that Bring You Peace

This could be anything from a cozy blanket or cup of tea to going for a run or sharing a yoga class with your besties. The idea is to identify what settles you when everything feels like it's falling apart. What centers and grounds you? What are you subconsciously drawn to when you're anxious? How do you self-soothe?

My big 'ah-ha!' moment for this component was when my mind drifted over my craft room. I am a rather passionate crafter. Fiber art is my primary medium and I gleefully pick up new skills in working with fibers wherever I can. I like to create all sorts of things, some well-made, some not. Some aren't even finished and will be pulled apart in the future to make something else. The production isn't the point; the creation is.

Creating brings me back to my center. It settles my spirit and fills my heart with peace. Look to the activities or items that make you feel like yourself again, even when you haven't felt like much of anything to this point.

Your Village - Extended Edition

This final component is a big one, and it's where most people trip up and fall back into learned identities. In order to make this a little bit easier, let's jump back to Chapter 3 and look at who you identified as the people in your village. Certainly, the people who are closest to you right now belong in this area. This is an excellent starting point.

There may also be people who have passed out of your life, either through death or circumstances, to whom you still hold a deep emotional connection. Imagine for a moment that they were still in your life. Where in the relationship circles would they fall? Would they be a part of your village? Why or why not? Remember to *shed the should* here. This is not about who you were in relation to them, not about the identity you learned in this relationship dynamic. This is about how much of your story they would get to know and how dependable they would be.

Exercise 6: Field Notes

It's time to get out your favorite documenting tool and prepare to put it through some heavy lifting. If you're a write-in-the-book person like me, I strongly encourage you to go to my website and download the worksheet for this exercise. It will serve you well. And hey, if you print it out, you can always fold it in half and use it as a bookmark, right?

Put on your imaginary archaeologist hat (or, if you have a real one, go ahead and put that on too!) and get ready to catalog all of the components of you. Keep in mind:

🌿 Work through one component fully before moving on to the next. This will help you remain in the right mindset and may help you remember some things you otherwise would have forgotten.

117

🔥 Be as specific or generic as you like when cataloging. These are your field notes; you're in control of them. All that matters is that when you return to them, you know exactly what you meant and why you included something.

🔥 Capture as many pieces as come to mind. The more you have, the more clues you will uncover that lead to your core self.

🔥 This exercise is for your benefit alone; nobody will be reviewing your work, so the more honest you are with yourself, the more helpful the result will be.

Step 1:

Beginning with Personal Artifacts, create a list, documenting the name of each artifact in the component.

Step 2:

Examine the items carefully and describe them the way an archaeologist might.

Step 3:

Repeat with each component until all five have been completed.

When I worked through this cataloging process at the end of 2021, I had a deadline so I could teach this class. I had to rush through my lists a bit. You don't need to. The process can take as little or as much time as you need it to, so don't put artificial deadlines on yourself. You're unpotting here; be gentle and give yourself some extra nourishment and affirmation. You are doing good work!

8

THREADS MAKE THE TAPESTRY

It was two weeks before I was scheduled to teach this class on building a purpose board and I still wasn't ready. Frustrated and a little bit anxious, I settled into that same - now well-worn - ergonomic chair at my desk and studied a picture of an old woman in a recliner and a teenager kneeling next to her. They both smiled broadly. The old woman held a green and white afghan on her lap. They're clearly related; you can easily see it in their faces.

To most anyone, it would look like a basic family picture, one of a million that fills yellowing photo albums stuffed into bookcases, rarely remembered until an elder begins to reminisce. To me, it's a personal artifact.

The old woman is my great grandmother and the teenager is me. The blanket on her lap is the very first afghan I ever made, which I gifted her that year at Christmas. The truly special part about this image is that she had given me the yarn and the pattern for the afghan as a gift one year prior. It perfectly captures our relationship: the give-and-take we shared, the unconditional love and respect between the two of us.

This picture lives on my bedroom dresser where I can see it every day. She was my best friend and the first person to see me for me without trying to change me. She was everything magical about Christmas to me, and that magic she imbued in the holiday is why it was, and is, my favorite. I try now to bring that magic to Christmas for my own family to keep a bit of her with me every year.

"Breathe, Becca. Look at it closely. What is it missing? Tear it out and try again. Don't be afraid of tearing things out."

She also taught me to crochet. More than that – she taught me to create. How to look at an object, study its pieces, learn from those pieces, and incorporate something inspiring from them into my own work. How to envision something new and imagine the steps necessary to bring it into being out of nothing.

My great grandmother is one of the people on my list, too. She passed away when I was 16, and her presence was so impactful in my life that I can still hear her warm voice in my ear when I get frustrated that something isn't working the way I want it to. "Breathe, Becca. Look at it closely. What is it missing? Tear it out and try again. Don't be afraid of tearing things out." Her gift to me was wisdom that goes far beyond crocheting or creating.

As I immersed myself in the memory of that photograph and the waves of emotion flooded over me, I realized why all of my lists of clues mattered. Every single thing on those lists was connected. The things that are most important to my core self are found in each item, each experience, each person on my list. The threads were staring at me the whole time, just waiting for me to find them – to find myself.

The lists you created from your field notes in Chapter 7 hold clues to your core self, too. You've found all of your personal artifacts and described them. You've identified the things that bring you joy, peace, and pride and reveled in them. You've looked into your village and found the people who have helped you become who you are. There are themes, and there are threads embedded in those lists. You are so very close to knowing who your core self is and what your purpose is! You are holding the keys to your success in these lists.

Now, it's time to dig in and organize - and truly understand - what all of these pieces mean to your core self. As you work through the exercises in this chapter, breathe. Look closely – what's missing from the picture? If it doesn't make sense, tear it out and try again. Don't be afraid of tearing things out.

Exercise 7: Investigation

As with your field notes in Chapter 7, move through your components one by one. Start with whichever component draws you the most, and complete it before you move on to the next. It may be tempting to jump around between them, and I promise you will find more clarity in your connections by staying in one component until it is completed.

Step 1:

Review the first item in your chosen area and consider why it was worthy enough, among all of the things and experiences in your life, to land on your list.

- Is it connected to an event or an experience?

- What significance did that event or experience hold in your life?

For me, the photo with my great grandmother was set at Christmas. That was and continues to be my favorite time of year. I have so many good, warm, loving memories attached to Christmas, most of them involving her. After she passed, Christmas became kind of a dead spot in my memory until I had a family of my own to share that magic and love with.

Step 2:

Stay with the same item.

- Are there significant people connected with your item?

  - What role did they play in your life?

  - Was their presence impactful for you? How?

  - What feelings did that moment with that person inspire then, and what do you feel now when you think about it?

Clearly, the significant person attached to my photograph is my great-grandmother. She was my best friend, my mentor, and one of the few people who accepted me for me. I can see my pride in my own face in the photograph; the pride of being able to gift that particular project back to the person who guided me into this craft, knowing that it would fill her with the same pride. It was the best way I could come up with

126

to share a fraction of the love she'd poured into me back to her.

Step 3:

Continue with your item and think of one or two words that encompass everything you've already noted.

🌿 What is most important to express about this particular piece? Go with your instinct.

You're tapping into your core self here; listen to it and hear what it's trying to tell you. The two that came to mind instantly for my photograph were love and generosity.

That's a lot to think about. It may energize you; if so, keep going with your area. It may wear you out; in this case, give yourself some grace and rest before you tackle the next item. There's no due date on your process and no teacher to turn it in to. Come back to it when you're rested and ready to go again.

Exercise 8: Analysis

Once you have completed this process for every item you noted in all five areas, it's time to analyze. You may choose to do this in a chart, a word cloud, sticky notes, or any other method that works for you when you are organizing ideas.

Step 1:

Gather all of your distilled words from the last step of the process and sort them into like categories.

🌿 Where are the threads in your themes? Some may naturally go together, while others may seem to bridge categories. That's ok; do what makes sense to your brain.

Step 2:

As these clusters form, approach them with curiosity. Can you give your clusters a name?

🌿 Is there one word or idea that seems central to the others around it?

❧ Is there a larger theme that covers all of your clusters?

❧ What about the words between clusters; do they fit better with a named cluster now, or do they still tie ideas together to make them clearer?

❧ Is your bridging word a better name for both clusters?

The process you are going through right now is mapping your core self. You're learning the values that are most important to you and giving names to them. It may be uncomfortable, especially if you've never done an exercise like this before. You might be feeling a bit guilty about focusing on yourself so much. It's a lot easier to shove yourself into the background and focus on what other people need. That's the old pattern, though. That's the pot you've outgrown.

If you're feeling resistance as you work through the process, hop back over to Chapter 3 and remind yourself about how you can take care of your unpotted self. Take the time to be gentle with yourself and listen to what your needs are. Attend those needs while you're figuring out this new root structure, because that's exactly what this process is.

You are in a new place, full of nutrients you aren't sure how to locate yet. Your roots might be a bit tangled up, you don't have the comfort of your old structure to fall back on. Tap into the strategies you've created and lean on your village. You will find your way again, your roots will straighten, and you will be amazed at the abundance of nourishment you will find to help you grow even more.

Exercise 9: Distillation

Step 1:

Once you've worked through mapping, review the themes that rose to the top while you were naming your categories.

🌿 What jumps out at you?

🌿 Can you distill them down further?

There is no minimum or limit on the number of themes you can have, and distilling judiciously will make your work in the future easier. Three to five is a good range to aim for; one and two tend to be overly broad to the point that they're not helpful in our next step. More than five can make your job cumbersome and make you less likely to stick with the work ahead.

My mapping led me to three themes: justice, sharing, and love. These are my core self's values. Your themes are your core self's values. Absent all other roles you have taken on in your life, these are the things that are most important to the one and only you.

There's only one task left to define your purpose, and that is actually defining your purpose. You have done all of the pre-work necessary for this task. You have shed your learned roles. You have investigated your personal artifacts and all of the people, items, and experiences that are connected to your values. You have sifted, organized, and distilled those into words that define your core self's values.

You have done so much to get to this point. It's time to take the momentum of all of that effort and channel it into your purpose statement.

Exercise 10: Naming Your Why

I recommend you sit with your values to complete this task. Take some time to yourself. Grab a cup of coffee, tea, or whatever makes you feel warm and full. Get comfortable. Pamper yourself for a bit. Some light background noise is ok, though silence heavily encourages you to be centered and mindful of your thoughts.

Step 1:

Stew on these words, the themes you identified in Exercise 9.

- 🌿 Think about how they connect to how you have lived your life.

- 🌿 Think about how you want them to connect to your life.

🍃 Your purpose statement will begin to form in your mind. If it's right, you will feel more connected to it every day. If it's not, look for what's missing, tear it out, and start again.

🍃 If some of it works but there's a piece that doesn't seem to fit, leave that piece open for revision. The statement should be a simple statement, and you should have an understanding of what drives that statement. This is necessary to apply all of the work you've done to your daily life.

My purpose statement is, "Fight wisely, share freely, love recklessly." This means that I will fight for justice everywhere, and I will make sure the energy I put into those fights has the potential to effect change, however incremental. It means that I will share my excess resources (excess being the key word, because I must meet my own needs before I have the capacity to give any away) as freely as I can, to whomever is in need, whenever I can. My resources are not only material or financial; they include my time, my energy, my knowledge, and my wisdom.

It means that my actions will be rooted in love no matter who they are directed to, and I will pour out as much love as I possibly can with each action. How it is received by someone else is none of my business; my only requirement is to give the love. I will also receive the love of others when their actions are rooted in it. This is my purpose. This describes my core self. It is who I am.

Your purpose statement does not need to look like mine. You are a different person and only you can decide what yours is. What is most important is that when you have crafted it, the words sit right with your spirit and flow easily from your lips. You can speak it into a mirror, explain it, and say, "This is my purpose. This describes my core self. It is who I am."

rubedo

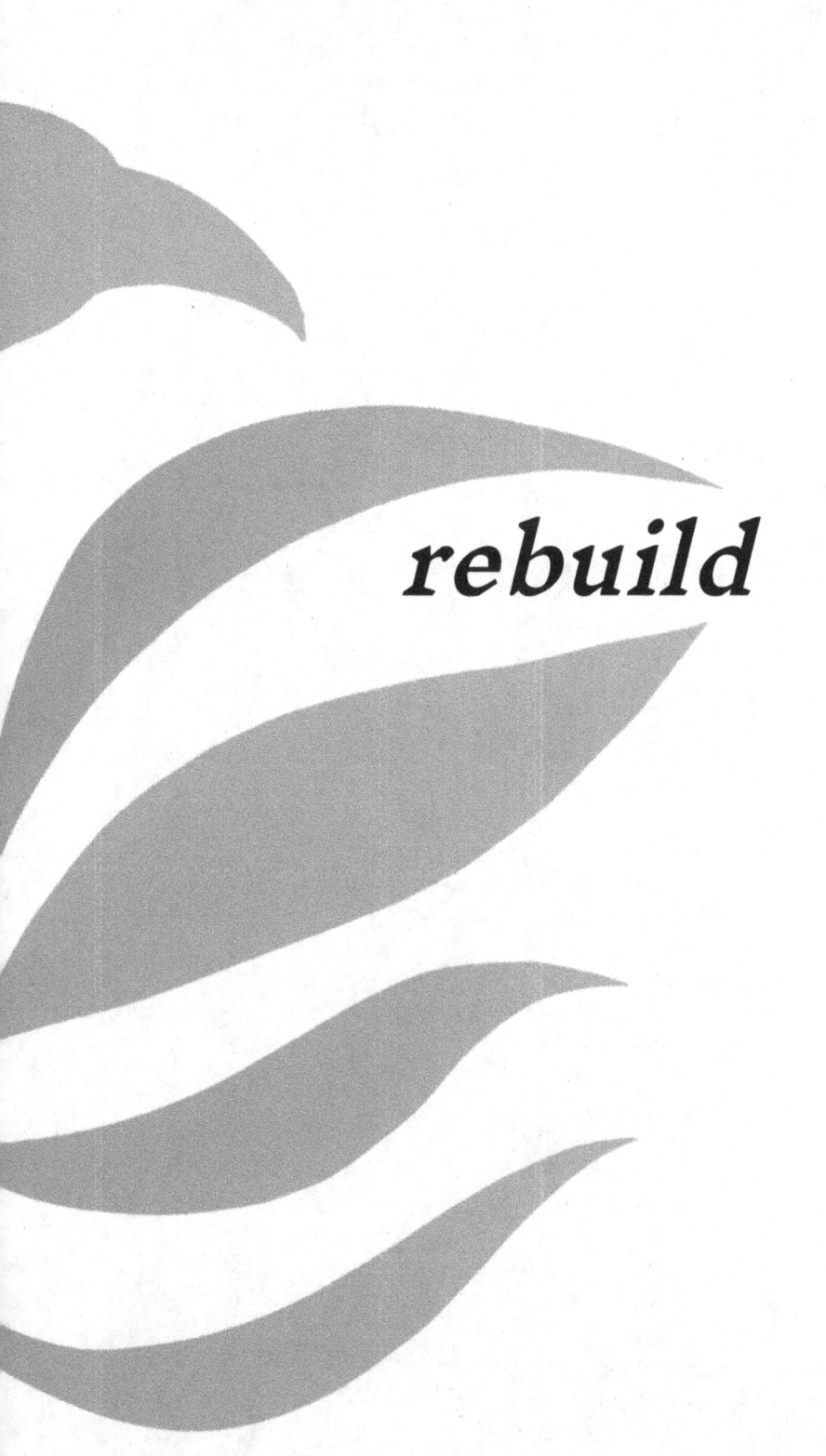

rebuild

9

HERE BE DRAGONS

You have your purpose statement! You know who your core self is, and you can describe yourself to the world! You have done some really heavy lifting and released the idea that your worth as a human is tied up in how much you do for someone else! Awesome, right? But...now what? How exactly do you apply this in your daily life so all of this work you've put yourself through actually provides the peace, freedom, and contentment you've been craving for so long? Lucky for you, I had enough coffee to write out the next steps in this chapter... and it was only mostly cold.

You have found your proverbial key. Your purpose, and the statement you've crafted alongside it, is your key that nobody can ever take from you. It's yours. A key is a portal to freedom, but only if you know where you're going.

How can you know where you're going if you've never been there? The first time you traveled to a place you'd never been on your own, did you just set out and hope you'd end up at the right place? Or did you tap into resources around you to understand the steps necessary to get from point A to point B? If I had to guess, you probably planned your route on at least a high level, noting key landmarks to guide you on your way. You probably used a map at some point during the process.

If you were to stop reading here, you would be setting off into the world with your precious key and no idea of where or how to go where you intend to. You have the tool, and it's not quite useful to you yet beyond the exhilaration of simply possessing something you've desired for a long time. Rather than stopping, though, take the time to do a little more planning to draw your map for how you will move through the world going forward.

This takes the form of learning how to align your actions and choices with your purpose statement and your understanding of what drives it. Your map isn't a picture of a country or a city. It is a schematic of your inner being, all of the infinite cosmos that make up the one unique you. It includes your learned identities as well as your core self because your learned identities should reflect how your core self shows up in the world. Pop back to Chapter 7 if you need a refresher on either the concepts of learned identities or your core self.

Your map is how you apply everything you've learned through this book so far to your daily life. You've already done the hard work in this process, and now you get to the fun part: learning how to draw the map and apply it. This is how you will effect lasting change, work through burnout (or keep from falling into that pit), and buffer yourself from relapse. As you draw this map, your purpose statement becomes your lodestar, a guiding light, and that unchanging point in your sky that helps you find your way.

The process of drawing your map requires a fair amount of concentration and contemplation. You need a space that is exclusively yours to do this work in. You'll need it as you consult your map throughout your travels, too. Now is the time to create that space if you don't already have one.

Exercise 11: Haven Sweet Haven

Step 1:

Identify a space in your home that you can claim as yours and yours alone. It's not shared with a child, a spouse, a roommate, or a pet. You can invite them in from time to time, but they have no right to that space without your invitation. This is especially challenging to do when you are used to accommodating others. Remember, though, you have the right to take up space! This may be logistically easier for some than for others. If you cannot claim an entire room for yourself, find a corner of a room that is yours alone.

Step 2:

Once you've identified your space, set boundaries around it. These boundaries can be physical and verbal.

- Place a privacy screen between your corner and the rest of the room.

- Close the door if you have an entire room and place a "do not disturb" sign on the outside.

142

State your boundaries to those you share your living space with.

🌿 Let them know what cues to look for to know when you are not to be disturbed or, conversely, when you are open to having them join you in your space. Then, enforce those boundaries.

🌿 When someone does not respect the cues you have communicated, gently and firmly remind them of the boundary and why it exists. They'll catch on, and your space will feel more and more like your retreat.

Step 3:

Decorate your space. It should be a calm place to exist and contain reminders of who your core self is.

🌿 If you have room, it may be time to pull some of the personal artifacts you identified during your work in Chapter 7 out. Choose pieces that elicit strong emotional responses when you look at them and place them where they can catch your eye and remind you of your purpose.

❧ Go through your lists of things that bring you joy, pride, and peace to help fill this space. When you enter it, you want to feel your learned identities falling away as you step fully into your core self. This is a space for you – just you – to exist.

One tool you can leverage to maximize your use of space, include events or feelings that you don't have artifacts for, or pull a sense of your exclusive space into another place – perhaps where you do your daily work – is a purpose board. I've mentioned this before in passing; it's essentially a vision board but for your why instead of for your what. It can be electronic or physical. Electronic versions serve well as computer desktop backgrounds, while physical versions take the form of art in your space.

- As you are creating your purpose board, think about what will be most effective in reminding you of your purpose and purpose statement. You want this piece to be effective in helping you *shed the should* on a regular basis and transporting you to a place where you can connect with your core self for consultation.

My purpose board has my purpose statement (Fight Wisely, Share Freely, Love Recklessly) across the top, with images below that bring to my mind those intended feelings and values. Of course, the picture of me kneeling next to my great grandmother is on my board. It is part of a collage that fills me with peace, joy, and contentment. My board reflects me back to myself, as yours should do for you. This is your mirror for your core self; look and marvel in it regularly.

With your space established and decorated, you are now ready to draw your map. This is a big process, and you have handled big processes already. The exercises you worked through as you walked this journey have trained your muscles to do this heavy lifting. This is the level-up, and you're ready for it.

There are five steps to this mapping process.

Inventory

List out all of your obvious learned identities - those roles you were socialized into that define your relationship to someone else, like spouse, parent, coworker, friend, etc.

Extrapolate

Parse out more subtle learned identities where the obvious ones intersect or overlap. These may also appear when the obvious one means different things in different contexts, like your employee identity when you hold two jobs with very different cultures.

Assess

Does each of these learned identities - and how you express them - align with your purpose statement? If so, great. If not, where and how does change need to happen? Are you holding onto a *what*?

Define Done

Imagine a future where you have let go of any *whats* that hold you back and have embraced your *why*. What does that look like for each identity that did not align with your purpose statement?

Plot Your Course

Develop incremental steps to go from point A (where you are today) to point B (the future you imagined for yourself in Step 4).

We'll walk through them in more detail together, one by one, in Exercise 12.

WARNING

This is Expert Level. Do not, under any circumstances, attempt Exercise 12 unless you have worked through and completed Exercises 1-11. Those eleven exercises are designed to prepare you for this next major step in your journey. If you are simply reading through the book right now, skip ahead to Chapter 10 and come back to this point after you have completed your work in full.

If you are ready to proceed, take this one step at a time. It's not called Expert Level for nothing. One way to envision the process you're about to master is like learning to solve a speed cube. You know the ones, six-sided with nine blocks of colored stickers on each side. It feels impossible at first glance, and the first couple goes at it may be frustrating - right up until you realize that the solution is a pattern.

This is a pattern, too. It might feel impossible at first glance, and the pattern is right there, waiting for you to click into it. Take a deep breath, work through it deliberately, and you will amaze yourself. I'll be right here as your biggest cheerleader with a huge grin on my face when you finish it.

Exercise 12: Your Personal Treasure Map

In this exercise, you get to draw a map that represents all of your personal complexity. You have spent a lot of time focusing on your core self – and rightfully so! Now, it's time to pull back and fold your learned identities back into your work.

Keep an extra watchful eye out for 'shoulds' creeping into your process here. Approach this part of your work like an anthropologist, with curiosity and without judgment.

I very strongly recommend that you grab the free worksheets for this exercise from my website. It will simplify things significantly for you!

Step 1: Inventory

Learned Identity Name	Primary Environment	Interacts With (People)	Restricted In:		
			Behavior?	Language?	Dress?
Spouse	Home	Partner	Minimal	No	No
Parent	Home	Children	Moderate – have to be a good example	Moderate – no profanity, age appropriate words	Minimal – must cover important bits
Employee	Office	Coworkers Manager Team members	Moderate – professional standards	Significant – no profanity, professional jargon	Business casual

Think about your learned identities and create a list of them similar to the field notes you created in Chapter 7. The more identities you are able to plot out, the more informative your map will be. If it's overwhelming to list all of them, start with the ones that have the largest impacts in your life. These tend to fall into three categories: work, family, and social.

§ Name them.

§ Identify the primary environments in which they exist.

§ Identify the people they interact with or have responsibility toward.

Question each identity.

🌀 Is its role a socially restricted one?

🌀 How is it restricted in:

   🌀 Behavior?

   🌀 Language?

   🌀 Dress?

Note these answers as well as whether this identity may take precedence over another if they were to intersect.

🌀 Think about the example of bringing a partner to a work-sponsored holiday party. Which identity is going to be dominant in that situation?

   🌀 How?

   🌀 Why?

There are no right or wrong answers in your inventory. Be honest with your reality so you can make a frank assessment.

Step 2: Extrapolate

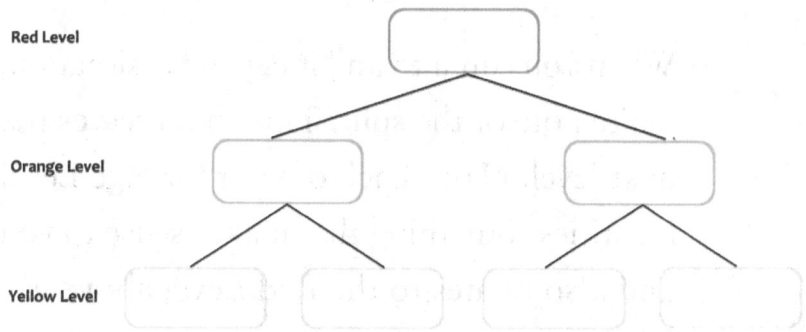

Red Level

Orange Level

Yellow Level

As you work through your identities, you may notice a tendency to say, "Well, it depends on the situation." And you're right – it absolutely does! You have layers of identities within these learned ones that express how you adapted to various situations you've been presented with. When you're drawing a map, though, you don't start with the detail and work out. You start with the largest known quantity and work your way down to the finer points that help a traveler navigate their path. Do the same thing here.

A quick note: I'll be using rainbow colors to help clarify which layer we're talking about at each point. You will find rainbow layers of identities in some, not in others – that's ok. Working through Step 1 found your Red Level learned identities.

⚘ Dig into one of your Red Level learned identities a bit.

  ⚘ When you run into an "it depends" situation, make note of the split. This split creates the next level. Name each of your Orange Level identities something that makes sense to you and also relates to the Red Level above it.

  ⚘ Repeat this process with each identity named in the Orange Level, and then so on until you don't have any more "it depends" situations. Add colors to the end of the rainbow if you need to. Go with your instincts on this; if it feels like the end, it's the end.

⚘ Add all of your newly-named learned identities to your inventory chart.

⚘ For each identity you name, regardless of the level, follow the exploration method outlined in Step 1.

Your map is really starting to come together! You now have an inventory of your complexity and how your different identities interplay with one another. It's kind of awe-inspiring to be exposed to that picture, like knowing a mountain range exists and then being 40,000 feet high and seeing it laid out before you. That view gives you the opportunity to assess where you are right now, at this very moment. You can't develop a plan to move forward without a starting point; you need a point A to figure out how to get to point B.

Step 3: Assess

Now is the time to integrate your purpose and purpose statement into the map creation process. Holding your identities and how they present to the world up to the light of your purpose will give you a very clear image of your point A.

※ Choose an identity rainbow and begin at the Red Level. Review what you've noted about potential restrictions and interactions, both with other identities and with other people.

   ※ Does it align with your purpose?

   ※ If not, why?

   ※ If so, take note of explicitly how it aligns.

🌿 Walk down through the levels of that identity and make the same assessment for each.

🌿 Does it align with your core self?

🌿 Why or why not?

🌿 Is there a *what* that you need to let go of?

🌿 Repeat this process for each identity rainbow. Remember to include all of your Red Levels, even those that don't have any other colors with them.

Step 4: Define Done

Once you've completed your assessment, review your work. Are there obvious areas that need to change? Nonalignment areas tend to cluster along with a few scattered outliers. Hone in on the clusters first; those signal where major changes need to happen in order to bring your learned identities into alignment with your purpose, your core self.

Pay attention here: these areas are where you are most likely to develop burnout. This is where you are holding onto the whats that keep you chained to the old way of thinking that you've already moved

154

beyond. Name those whats. Call them out and don't let them hide behind the mirage. Bring them into your purpose's light.

Don't forget to go back and address the outliers, too. That doesn't mean you have to solve everything immediately; it means you need to decide on incremental steps to pull yourself back into alignment. Before you chart those steps, figure out what done looks like.

- What would alignment for the Red Level of that identity include for you? Dream about it a little, and don't be afraid to dream big. Everything big is done in bite sized pieces, so don't shortchange yourself by minimizing your done.

- Now, imagine that you are in that place with that identity. How does that single change ripple through the rest of the levels?

  - Are there still identities that would need attention, or does that change mitigate all of the places that are misaligned?

155

🌸 For each remaining point of misalignment, decide what done looks like. How do you want to exist in that space?

There are no right or wrong answers here either. This is your life, you don't have to cater it to anyone's specific vision of how you should behave. *Shed the should* and trust your gut.

Step 5: Plot Your Course

You have point A, you have point B. How do you get from one to the other? What incremental steps are necessary to make that crossing?

🌸 Start with the big changes that need to happen.

   🌸 What are the barriers you see?

   🌸 What choices do you need to make to overcome (or go around) them?

   🌸 Evaluate dependencies in your steps. Which step needs to happen before another so you can progress? Make sure they are small enough that you can visualize progress and large enough that tracking that progress doesn't feel like a chore.

- ❦ If one is too big, break that one down and find something in the middle.

- ❦ If they're too small and your course looks overwhelming, combine some. Don't break it down to the level of some online mapping programs that tell you to pull out of your driveway before you begin your trip.

Each of your steps will align with some sort of action. Actions must align with your purpose and purpose statement to keep you on the path toward personal freedom. As you're planning your course, evaluate the actions you need to take at each step and ensure that they also align with your purpose. Make sure you're not turning South on a road when you need to turn North.

Your purpose is a lodestar, a point in the sky on which to stay focused. Each step should bring you closer to that purpose. If it doesn't, why are you doing it? Is there another way to produce the same result while staying aligned with your purpose?

If you find yourself struggling at any point in this process, check in with your village. Look back to Chapter 3 if you need a reminder of who's in your village. You may want to work through that exercise again if you think your village has evolved since you last reviewed it.

Remember that these are the people who know you best; they know the most about your story, and they are there for you when you need them. They will tell you the things you need to hear, even if you don't want to listen to them, because they love you. They can provide the insight you need to progress through your block. Also, they want to. Let them. Give them the gift of being allowed to help.

The first time through this mapping process is always the hardest because it involves a *lot* of cataloging and analysis. Now that you've been through it once, it will be easier moving forward – you only need to do steps

3 through 5 as maintenance. They'll also go much faster because you only need to note where things have changed. Always come back to whether you are in alignment with your purpose.

Exercise 13: Rituals Are Not Luxuries

Now is a perfect time to establish some rituals around your assessment process. This is where that lovely space you created for yourself really benefits you.

Tap into your senses and use the things that bring you joy and peace to define steps that will get you in the headspace to work through this assessment each time you work through it.

- Engage your taste with a favorite beverage

- Activate your touch with a soft blanket or comfortable chair

- Pique your sense of smell by lighting a candle or melting some scented wax

- Soothe your sight by adjusting the lighting

❧ Turn on music – or not – to meet your mind's sound needs

Set the mood for focusing on you, and then delve into the process.

Your ritual doesn't have to be super involved, either. Take one or two actions that feel comfortable and natural to you, whatever will spur your brain to get into assessment mode, and do them every time you sit down in your personal space to review your map. The more you do this, the faster your mind will associate those actions with slipping into assessment.

Creating and reinforcing a ritual when you are in a strong and firm place gives you an easy entry to this meditative space when you start responding to the world in an emotional way because your brain is fatigued.

You and I both know that putting words on paper to work in real life is not always as easy as it sounds. This mindset shift that you have made is still very new – a

160

seedling you've transplanted that needs to be protected and nurtured. Reading a book and following exercises can only take you so far if you don't put protective wards around the new growth.

The old mindset – the old pot and all the weeds that come along with it – still exists in your head. You know it's not useful. You know it's too small for your growth. It will still call to you, and because it's familiar, that call will sometimes be strong.

When you find yourself arguing with that old pot, enter your rituals. Remind yourself of who you are, where you are, where you're going, and how you're going to get there. Your purpose is your power. Surrender to its loving, healing energy and witness how the *what* that you've operated under for so long yields to the light of your *why*.

10

INTO YOUR UNKNOWN

I'd like you to step back for a moment. Go to the exercises you did in Chapters 4 and 6. Reread what your answers were, then take some time to reflect on them. Now that you've completed this process, how have your answers evolved?

As you've worked through this book, you've done a lot of hard work. You followed along with the exercises I laid out. You encountered pieces of you that likely weren't so comfortable to address. You unpotted yourself, maybe once, maybe several times.

You tapped into your village to help you work through the tough spots and found your way through. You released the idea that your value is tied to your productivity, and you replaced it with the assured

163

knowledge that your value is an intrinsic part of your being. You embraced your core self without the weight of others' expectations. You defined your personal purpose statement, succinctly describing that core self to the world. You learned how to use your purpose to guide you through the ups and downs of life.

You no longer allow someone else to tell you what success should look like. You know what it looks like because you define it for yourself every day. You have a radically different view of yourself and how you move through the world compared to when you cracked the cover, and now you're close to turning the last page.

But you haven't reached the end.

You might be thinking, "Hold up, you promised me that by the time I was done reading I'd be good!" Here's the key: the end of this book is not the end of your process. Just like your understanding of yourself and the world has evolved through the time it took you to read this book, it will continue to evolve long after you lay it down. You will continue to evolve.

This process is not a one-and-done. Rather, it is a structure you can return to over and over as you learn more about yourself and the world. You will continue to grow; your purpose must necessarily grow with you.

Redefining your purpose will happen multiple times throughout your life. Your purpose statement will shift. It won't always happen in a linear way. I encourage you to have this book and your work nearby to revisit often and remind yourself of why you ended up where you did. I encourage you equally to be willing to release your conclusions; they are based on the you who exists today. Tomorrow's you will know more.

You are going to form new relationships, experience new things, bring new ideas into reality. As you do, you will develop new perspectives. Some of those perspectives will connect to what you have already assessed. Some will be focused on things you have not yet encountered. All of it is relevant to the totality that is you.

As you walk through those adventures and find new perspectives, you will experience friction. Friction is unavoidable in our lives, and you get to decide how you navigate it. Friction is a sign to pause and pay attention to what is going on. Something isn't sitting right.

When you feel that uncomfortable rubbing in your soul, stop. Breathe. Look closely – what is missing from the picture? If you can't readily identify where the issue is by holding it up to your purpose, it may be time to tear your purpose statement out and try again. Don't be afraid to tear things out.

Tearing out your work and trying again doesn't mean you're disposing of all of the effort that came before. Instead, you are starting with a blank slate from a place of experience. The process outlined in this book can be used over and over again... and it should be! From releasing old mindsets that pull you out of your alignment through redefining your purpose, each time you walk the path, it will become more familiar, and you will navigate it more quickly and with greater ease.

Mistakes are how humans learn, and those imperfections add an untamed artistry to the landscape you have built around you.

You will get to a point where you won't need to walk the whole path as you reassess your core self because you'll know where to go to target the friction you're

166

experiencing. It likely won't bring you to the same place twice. You're a human who values growth, so would you really want it to?

Once you lay each of those paths end to end, you'll discover a glorious journey with dotted periodic rest stops. The rest stops are necessary, but they're not the interesting part; the paths themselves are where joy and beauty revel. The journey you view from the eagle's perch will be filled with imperfections because you are human. Mistakes are how humans learn, and those imperfections add an untamed artistry to the landscape you have built around you.

Each time you reassess your core self and your purpose statement, begin by flying to that eagle's perch and taking in the totality of your journey so far. See where you have chosen to dip back into the ocean to gain some new understanding or gain a skill you need to keep going. Notice that there are no circles you've pushed around; the journey may be winding, but it is always moving forward.

Bask in the ease with which you've made choices because an option did – or didn't – align with your purpose. Take in the sumptuous, open sky above, blazing with the radiance and splendor of the northern lights, knowing each of your choices fed those undulating beams that illuminate the path forward.

Your life is not a destination but a journey full of exquisite scenery and wild, precipice curves. You've now drawn your map, and you finally hold the keys.

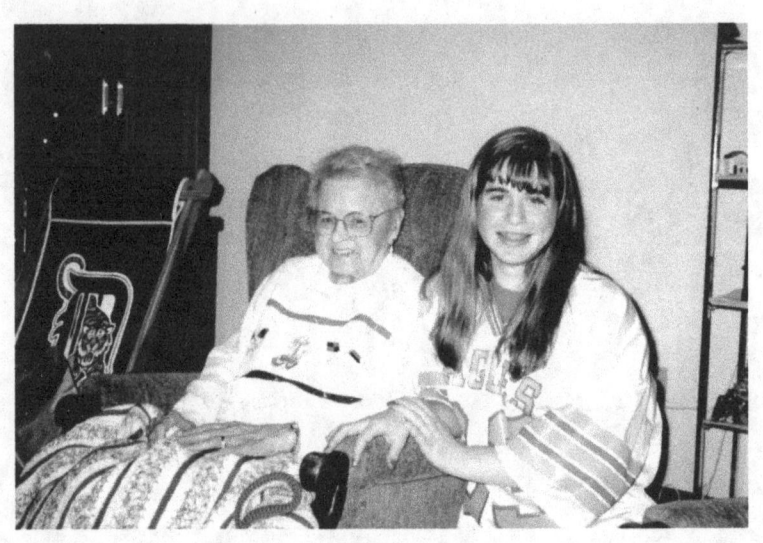

Acknowledgements

This book was written on the ancestral homelands of the **Meskwaki (Sauk & Fox), Myaamia, Očhéthi Šakówiŋ (Sioux), Hoocąk (Ho-Chunk), and Kiikaapoi (Kickapoo)** people. Indigenous peoples, including members of some of these nations, still live and practice their teachings and cultures here today. I honor these stewards of the lands and work to learn their history, much of which is excluded from our education. I encourage you to take the time to learn about the people whose homelands you live in.

A big shoutout goes to my **husband** and **children**, who delivered meals, endless hugs, and encouragement through the highs and lows of this process. This book is as much yours as it is mine. I love you always, to Pluto and back.

Gratitude to **Nicole** and **Darlene** for always having the right questions, whether to get me going or get me through the messy bits. Also, for evening chats, Saturday morning silliness, and a beautiful community.

To **Jen** and **Brenay**, two of the best sisters a girl could ask for. Whether I needed love, wise counsel, or boundless creativity, I knew either one of you would be willing to dive in. This book would be a pale shadow of itself without both of you.

Thanks to **Josh**, whose esoteric knowledge and associative abilities provided a framework for concepts in this book. It's easy to tie things together when there's a theme that fits so neatly.

Deep love and appreciation to **Dawn** and **Jess** for keeping me grounded and reminding me of my power. Also for silly memes and videos, screaming into the void, and upside down couch selfies.

To **Lara,** for being a role model and fellow traveler on this journey. There were a lot of bumps, curves, and swerves, but we did it. We figured it out!

To **Doreen,** for showing me how to conquer my own fear by being fearlessly yourself. Your beautiful friendship inspires me. I'll need your autograph once your book is done... maybe over lunch?

Everlasting gratitude to **Kelly,** for walking side by side with me through the garbage. And for helping me learn that it's ok to put myself first sometimes.

Eternal thanks to **Amanda,** who gave me permission to make mistakes. I'd still follow you anywhere. You're an amazing leader, and the world would be a better place with more like you.

High honors and adulation to **Luvvie Ajayi Jones,** whose writing gave me the kick in the pants I needed to stop making excuses and get up to do the thing. Also, for building a community filled with some of the greatest women I've ever known.

And finally, to the cousins. **Carla, Tracy, Kiesha, Val, Marcia, Camille, Sylvia, Elise, Joanna, Katy, Felicia, Oluwatoyin, Erika,** and probably a whole bunch more that aren't coming to mind at the moment but whom I cherish not even a little bit less. You are amazing. You inspire me with your intelligence, kindness, wit, and passion. I am so grateful for all of the time we've spent together, and can't wait for all of the adventures ahead. I want to be every single one of you when I grow up!

Rebecca Claeys is a wisdom steward and purpose coach helping professional women and gender nonconforming people experiencing personal friction claim peace and fulfillment in their lives. She is the creator of the Soul Alchemy Cycle and founder of Cleopatra's Seeds.

Rebecca is a Bachelor's educated Registered Nurse and holds credentials as a Certified Professional Coder and a Certified Program Integrity Professional. She has received numerous accolades for her work during the COVID-19 public health emergency, including a Certificate of Recognition and a Challenge Coin from the State of Wisconsin Department of Health Services and a Certificate of Appreciation from the US Army 78th Training Division.

After running on the corporate hamster wheel for 20 years chasing the next big career step (what she calls 'a what'), Rebecca now helps women and gender nonconforming professionals facing burnout to reclaim their root purpose (what she refers to as 'a why') so they define their freedom, joy, and success on their terms. Connect with her at

www.CleopatrasSeeds.com.

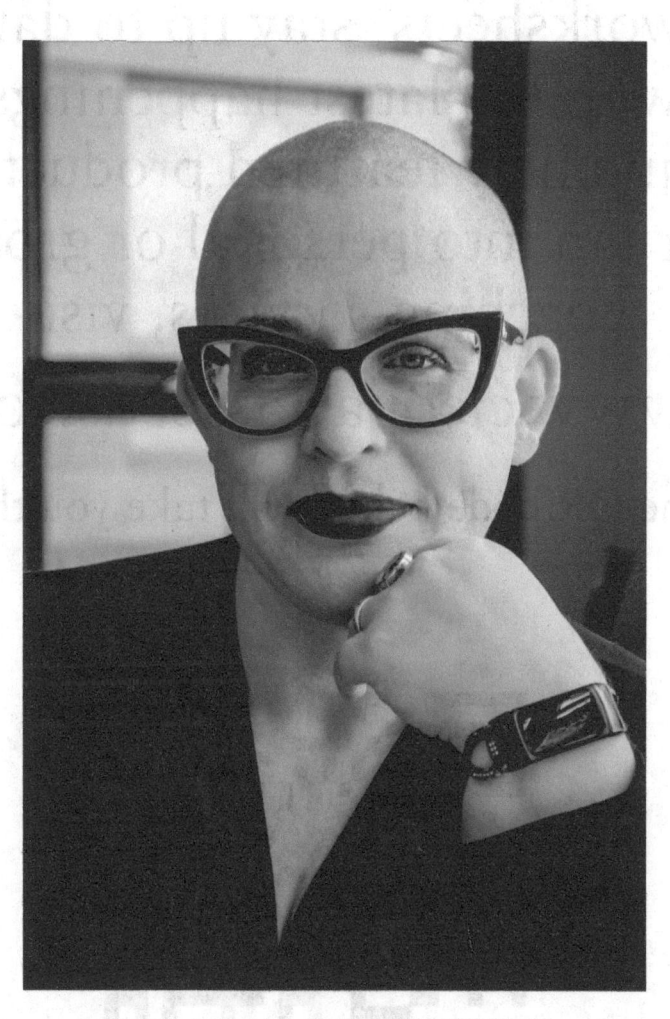

To access free exercise worksheets, stay up to date with the latest happenings, find new featured products, or tap into personal or group coaching services, visit

www.cleopatrasseeds.com

(the QR code below will take you there)